Radiation
Protection

Radiation Protection

STEWART C. BUSHONG, Sc.D., F.A.C.R., F.A.C.M.P.

Professor of Radiologic Science
Department of Radiology
Baylor College of Medicine
Houston, Texas

ESSENTIALS OF MEDICAL IMAGING SERIES

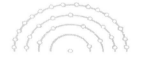

McGraw-Hill

Health Professions Division

New York   St. Louis   San Francisco   Auckland   Bogotá   Caracas   Lisbon   London   Madrid
Mexico City   Milan   Montreal   New Delhi   San Juan
Singapore   Sydney   Tokyo   Toronto

McGraw-Hill

A Division of The **McGraw·Hill** Companies

RADIATION PROTECTION

Essentials of Medical Imaging Series

1 2 3 4 5 6 7 8 9 0   MALMAL   9 9 8

ISBN 0-07-012013-7

This book was set in Berkeley by V&M Graphics.
The editors were John J. Dolan and Peter McCurdy.
The production supervisor was Heather A. Barry.
The text designer was Jose R. Fonfrias.
The cover designer was Robert Freese.
Malloy Lithographing, Inc. was printer and binder.

This book is printed on acid-free paper.

Visit The McGraw-Hill Health Professions Website at
http://www.mghmedical.com

Cataloging-in-Publication data is on file for this title at the Library of
Congress.

Dedicated to:

Bettie,
Leslie,
Stephen,
Andrew,
Butterscotch,[†]
Jemimah,[†]
Geraldine,[†]
Casper,[†]
Ginger,[†]
Sebastian,[†]
Buffy,[†]
Brie,[†]
Linus,[†]
Midnight,[†]
Boef,[†]
Cassie,[†]
Lucy,[†]
Toto,[†]
Choco,[†]
Molly,[†]
Maxwell[†]*and my lenses,*
Bandit,[†]
Kate,[†]
Misty,[†]
Chester,[†]
Petra,[†]
Travis,[†]
Ebony,[†]
April,[†] *and Cory*[†]

Contents

PREFACE   ix

CHAPTER 1

PROPERTIES OF MATTER AND ENERGY   1

CHAPTER 2

PROPERTIES OF RADIATION   9

CHAPTER 3

MEASUREMENT UNITS OF IONIZING RADIATION   17

CHAPTER 4

SOURCES OF IONIZING RADIATION   23

CHAPTER 5

BIOLOGICAL EFFECTS OF IONIZING RADIATION   29

CHAPTER 6

PATIENT RADIATION CONTROL   53

CHAPTER 7

OCCUPATIONAL RADIATION CONTROL   67

CHAPTER 8

RECOMMENDED RADIATION DOSE LIMITS   75

CHAPTER 9

SPECIALTY AREAS OF MEDICAL IMAGING   93

Nuclear Medicine Imaging   93

Diagnostic Ultrasound Imaging   97

Magnetic Resonance Imaging   101

APPENDIX A

GLOSSARY   119

APPENDIX B

APPROPRIATE TEXTBOOKS   133

APPENDIX C

ANSWERS   134

APPENDIX D

ADDITIONAL RESOURCES   137

Preface

IMAGING SCIENCE has changed considerably over the past twenty years. These changes have brought an incredible increase in information, understanding, and innovation. One result is that today, imaging technologists, medical physicists and physicians must know far more than their predecessors. The fund of knowledge required of these health professionals, especially the imaging technologist, for any of the qualifying examinations is so vast that the demands on learning and teaching are considerable.

Accompanying this expansion of knowledge are substantial changes in our occupational opportunities. Limited licensure, cross-training, and job splitting are changing the required competence and responsibilities of the imaging technologist. The principle focus of these occupational changes is to obtain more production with fewer employees. Managed healthcare will continue to exert economic and occupational restrictions on the imaging technologist.

This book is one in a series designed to make the learning process easier for the imaging technologist. Patient and operator protection are important in all areas of imaging technology. Consequently, the educator and student will find Volume 1 of this series useful regardless of the areas of specialization. The additional volumes concentrate on specialty topics and areas of examination.

None of these volumes is a textbook. Sometimes, especially when preparing for an examination, it is easier to commit statements of fact to memory while working with other sources to gain a better understanding of those facts. Each of these volumes contain extensive statements of fact that the author believes are essential for satisfactory completion of the respective qualification examination. These volumes are well illustrated because, as has been said, "A picture is worth a thousand words." Where graphs, charts or tables are included, they are accompanied by brief statements of fact. At the end of each chapter, there are practice questions patterned after the respective qualification examinations, such as the ABR, the ABMP, ARDMS, the CNMT and especially the ARRT and its subspecialty exams in mammography, computed tomography, angiointerventional procedures, and magnetic resonance imaging. Most examination panels, especially the ARRT, principally use Type A questions: a statement or stem followed by three incorrect answers and one correct answer. Type K questions are used less frequently. These contain multiple statements and the candidate selects the correct combination of answers. The practice questions provided here are of both types.

At the end of each volume, there are four appendices that the student and educator will find particularly helpful. Appendix A is a rather complete glossary of terms employed in imaging science and imaging technology. Appendix B lists the latest textbook publications covering the respective information areas of the volume. Appendix C contains the answers to the practice questions. Finally, Appendix D, Additional Resources, identifies sources of educational material covering the topics of the book. Here the student will find exceptional literature references to aid in understanding through additional reading of a particular subject. The educator will find this section helpful when assigning special topics or special projects to students.

Medical imaging as practiced today in all of its forms is based on special principles of physics. To many students, physics is the most feared of subjects. It does not have to be. The purpose of this volume is to ease that learning process, prepare the student for examination, and help to make physics fun.

STEWART C. BUSHONG, Sc.D., F.A.C.R., F.A.C.M.P.

Radiation Protection

Properties of Matter and Energy

- Atoms are not the smallest units of matter, but they are very important to radiology.

- An atom has two principal parts, a nucleus and an electron cloud, arranged similarly to the planets in the solar system.

- Only electrons are found in the electron cloud.

- Neutrons and protons, called **nucleons**, are found in the nucleus.

- The nucleus is about the same size as an electron but has much more mass.

- Each nucleon is composed of quarks which are held together by gluons.

- There are over 100 subnuclear particles. Only nucleons are important to radiology.

- An atom consists mostly of empty space.

- In an electrically neutral atom, the number of electrons in the electron cloud equals the number of protons in the nucleus.

- In an ionized atom, there is one less electron in the electron cloud.

- Electrons are arranged in precise orbits or energy levels.

- Electrons in orbits nearer the nucleus are more tightly bound.

- Outer-shell electrons are very loosely bound and therefore easily removed—**ionized**.

- Electron binding energy is measured in electron volts (eV).

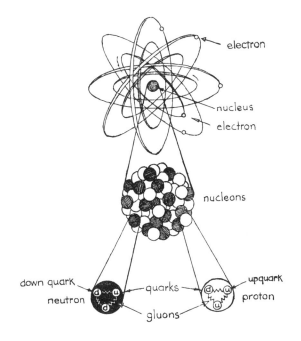

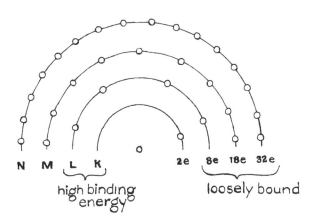

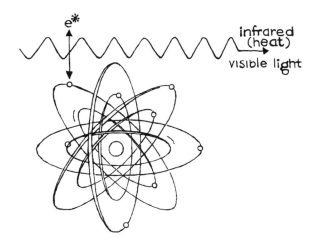

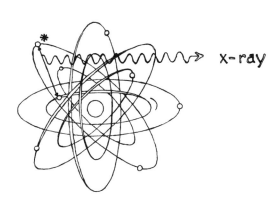

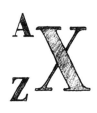

$$_Z^A X$$

e.g. $_{42}^{98}\text{Mo},\ _{43}^{99}\text{Tc},\ _{53}^{131}\text{I},\ _{74}^{184}\text{W},\ _{92}^{238}\text{Y}$

- Electrons are attracted to the nucleus by an electrostatic force. They remain in orbit because of centrifugal force.

- The electrostatic force of attraction for any electron equals the centrifugal force of repulsion.

- When electrons are caused to move from an inner to an outer orbit, or to an excited state, electromagnetic radiation is emitted when they return.

- When electrons in outer orbits change shells, the result is heat (infrared radiation) and/or visible light.

- When electrons in inner orbits of elements with high atomic number change shells, the result is x-ray emission.

- Some atoms have unstable nuclei and in order to become stable emit radiation, that is, radioactivity.

- The **atomic number** of an atom is the number of protons in its nucleus. Atomic number is indicated by Z.

- The **atomic mass** of an atom is the sum of the number of protons and the number of neutrons in its nucleus. Atomic mass is symbolized by A.

- In the designation for an atom, the atomic mass is a superscript preceding the chemical symbol, and the atomic number is a subscript preceding the chemical symbol.

- Atoms having nuclei with even numbers of protons and even numbers of neutrons are very likely to be stable. An odd number of protons and neutrons is associated with radioactivity.

- All atoms of the same element have the same atomic number.

- Atoms having the same atomic number are called **isotopes**.

- Atoms having the same number of neutrons are called **isotones**.

- Atoms having the same atomic mass are called **isobars**.

- Atoms having the same atomic number and atomic mass but different nuclear energy states are called **isomers**.

- Elements can have many isotopes, some stable and some radioactive.

Chapter 1 Practice Questions

1. Which of the following is the smallest?

   a. an atom
   b. an electron
   c. a molecule
   d. a compound

2. Which of the following is substantially the same for a nucleus and for an electron?

   1. energy
   2. mass
   3. charge
   4. velocity

   a. Only 1, 2, and 3 are correct.
   b. Only 1 and 3 are correct.
   c. Only 2 and 4 are correct.
   d. None are correct.

3. In an ionized atom, there is one less

   a. nucleon.
   b. proton.
   c. neutron.
   d. electron.

4. Which of the following has the highest binding energy?

   a. K-shell electrons
   b. L-shell electrons
   c. M-shell electrons
   d. O-shell electrons

5. Radioactivity is the process of

   a. a stable nucleus becoming unstable.
   b. an unstable nucleus becoming stable.
   c. an electron moving to an inner orbit.
   d. an electron moving to an outer orbit.

6. In the symbol $^{131}_{53}I$, the number 131 represents the

   a. atomic number.
   b. atomic mass.
   c. neutron number.
   d. electron number.

7. All atoms with the same atomic number are called

   a. isotopes.
   b. isotones.
   c. isobars.
   d. isomers.

8. An atom has two principal parts which are called

   a. electrons and molecules.
   b. molecules and compounds.
   c. compounds and nuclei.
   d. nucleus and electrons.

9. Electrons are
   a. organized inside the nucleus.
   b. arranged in orbits around the nucleus.
   c. usually bunched together.
   d. composed of neutrons and protons.

10. Which of the following is most likely involved in ionization?
    a. K-shell electrons   c. M-shell electrons
    b. L-shell electrons   d. O-shell electrons

11. Which of the following is associated with radioactivity?
    1. an unstable nucleus becoming stable
    2. removal of an electron
    3. emission of radiation
    4. ionization
    a. Only 1, 2, and 3 are correct.
    b. Only 1 and 3 are correct.
    c. Only 2 and 4 are correct.
    d. All are correct.

12. In the atomic notation $^{99m}_{42}$Tc, the 42 represents the
    a. atomic number.
    b. atomic mass.
    c. neutron number.
    d. electron number.

13. All atoms having the same number of neutrons are called
    a. isotopes.   c. isobars.
    b. isotones.   d. isomers.

14. Which of the following particles is a nucleon?
    1. nucleus   3. electron
    2. neutron   4. proton
    a. Only 1, 2, and 3 are correct.
    b. Only 1 and 3 are correct.
    c. Only 2 and 4 are correct.
    d. Only 4 is correct.

15. Which of the following is found in a nucleus?
    1. neutrons   3. gluons
    2. protons   4. quarks
    a. Only 1, 2, and 3 are correct.
    b. Only 1 and 3 are correct.
    c. Only 2 and 4 are correct.
    d. All are correct.

16. Electrons are positioned
    a. inside the nucleus.
    b. randomly outside the nucleus.
    c. both inside and outside the nucleus.
    d. in energy levels outside the nucleus.

17. Electrostatic force is that experienced by
    a. a human attracted to earth.
    b. a north pole attracted to a south pole.
    c. an electron attracted to a proton.
    d. a proton attracted to a neutron.

18. The number of protons in the nucleus of an atom is symbolized by
    a. A.
    b. B.
    c. X.
    d. Z.

19. In the following table of nuclear configurations, which is likely to be the most stable?

	Odd Number of Protons	Even Number of Protons
Odd number of neutrons	A	B
Even number of neutrons	C	D

    a. A
    b. B
    c. C
    d. D

20. All atoms having the same atomic mass are called
    a. isotopes.
    b. isotones.
    c. isobars.
    d. isomers.

21. Which of the following are found in the nucleus of an atom?
    1. nucleons
    2. neutrons
    3. protons
    4. electrons
    a. Only 1, 2 and 3 are correct.
    b. Only 1 and 3 are correct.
    c. Only 2 and 4 are correct.
    d. All are correct.

22. An atom can be described as being
    a. a dense mass.
    b. similar to the solar system.
    c. very unstable.
    d. easily disintegrated.

23. Which of the following types of electrons are most tightly bound to the nucleus?
    a. those inside the nucleus
    b. those closer to the nucleus
    c. those in the outer shells
    d. free electrons

24. Centrifugal force
    a. is similar to gravitational attraction.
    b. is the attraction of an electron to a proton.
    c. tends to keep rotating objects in a circular path.
    d. tends to cause rotating objects to go straight.

25. The number of protons in the nucleus of an atom is called the
   a. atomic number.
   b. atomic mass.
   c. nuclear number.
   d. electron number.

26. In the following table of nuclear configurations, which is likely to be the most unstable?

	Odd Number of Protons	Even Number of Protons
Odd number of neutrons	A	B
Even number of neutrons	C	D

   a. A
   b. B
   c. C
   d. D

27. All atoms having the same number of nucleons are called
   a. isotopes.
   b. isotones.
   c. isobars.
   d. isomers.

28. Which of the following is found outside the nucleus?
   a. neutron
   b. proton
   c. electron
   d. nucleon

29. An atom can be described as
   a. having low energy.
   b. consisting of mostly empty space.
   c. being spherical in shape.
   d. being very compact.

30. Which of the following electrons is most easily removed from an atom?
   a. those inside the nucleus
   b. those closer to the nucleus
   c. those in the outer shells
   d. free electrons

31. Electromagnetic radiation can be emitted when electrons
   a. are ejected from a nucleus.
   b. move from an inner shell to an outer shell.
   c. move from an outer shell to an inner shell.
   d. are removed from the atom.

32. The number of nucleons in an atom is symbolized by
   a. A.
   b. B.
   c. X.
   d. Z.

33. All atoms of the same element have the same number of
   a. nucleons.
   b. neutrons.
   c. protons.
   d. electrons.

34. Atoms having the same atomic number and atomic mass but different nuclear energy states are
    a. isotopes.   c. isobars.
    b. isotones.   d. isomers.

35. In order for an atom to be electrically neutral the number of
    a. protons must equal the number of neutrons.
    b. neutrons must equal the number of nucleons.
    c. nucleons must equal the number of electrons.
    d. electrons must equal the number of protons.

36. The tightness with which electrons are bound to the nucleus is expressed as electron binding energy, which is measured in
    a. joule (J).
    b. electron volt (eV).
    c. kilovolt peak (kVp).
    d. milliampere second (mAs).

37. Visible light results when
    a. electrons are absorbed by the nucleus.
    b. electrons are ejected from the nucleus.
    c. an electron in an outer orbit is excited and returns to that orbit.
    d. an electron in an inner orbit is removed and an outer-shell electron fills the void.

38. The number of nucleons in an atom is called the
    a. atomic number.   c. neutron number.
    b. atomic mass.   d. electron number.

39. All atoms of the same element have the same
    a. atomic number.   c. neutron number.
    b. atomic mass.   d. electron number.

40. Atoms having the same number of protons and neutrons but different nuclear energy states are called
    a. isotopes.   c. isobars.
    b. isotones.   d. isomers.

41. Which of the following are most tightly bound to a nucleus?
    a. K-shell electrons   c. M-shell electrons
    b. L-shell electrons   d. O-shell electrons

42. X rays are emitted when
    a. electrons are absorbed by the nucleus.
    b. electrons are ejected from the nucleus.
    c. an electron in an outer orbit is excited and returns to that orbit.
    d. an electron in an inner orbit is removed and an *outer-shell* electron fills the void.

43. All atoms with the same number of protons in the nucleus are called
    a. isotopes.   c. isobars.
    b. isotones.   d. isomers.

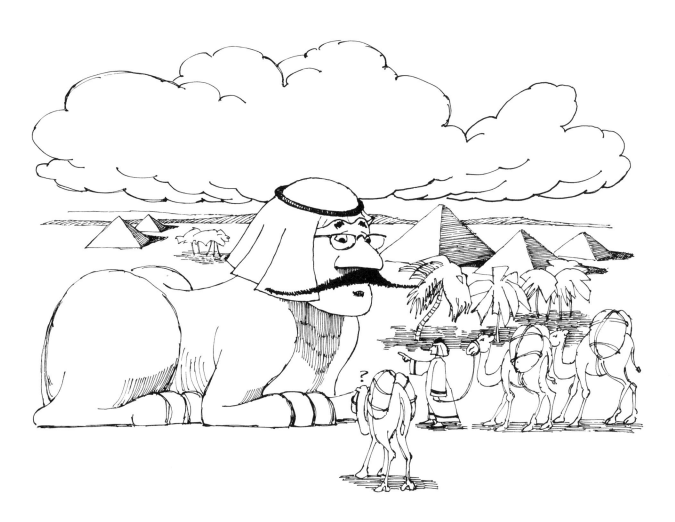

Properties of Radiation

- Radiation as used in medical imaging has two general forms—ionizing and nonionizing

IONIZING RADIATION

- X rays are used to form images in radiography, fluoroscopy, mammography, and computed tomography (CT).

- X rays are produced by machines. They are formed and emitted from the electron cloud of target atoms in an x-ray tube.

- γ rays are used to form images in nuclear medicine.

- γ rays are emitted from the nuclei of radio-active atoms.

- γ rays are emitted during radioactive decay.

NONIONIZING RADIATION

- Very high-frequency sound waves (ultrasound) are used to form diagnostic ultrasound images.

- The frequency range is 1 to 10 MHz.

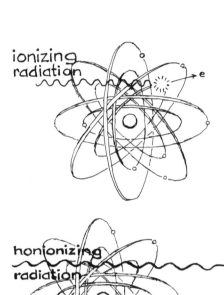

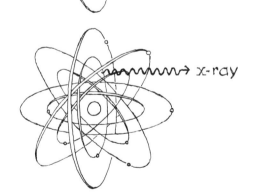

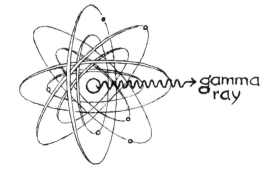

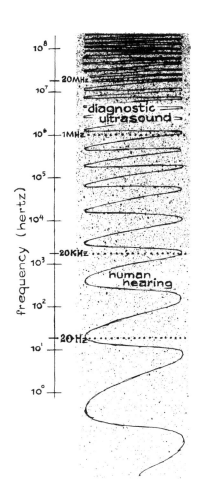

- The source of diagnostic ultrasound is a mechanically oscillating surface.

- Radio waves (radio frequencies, RF) are used in magnetic resonance imaging (MRI).

- The frequency range is 1 to 100 MHz.

- The source of RF is an oscillating electric current in a radio antenna.

PROPERTIES OF IONIZING RADIATION

- X and γ rays are electromagnetic radiation.

- Electromagnetic radiation consists of an electric field oscillating perpendicular to an oscillating magnetic field.

- Other forms of electromagnetic radiation are ultraviolet radiation (UV), visible light (VL), infrared radiation (IR), microwaves, and radio waves.

- Ultrasound is not electromagnetic.

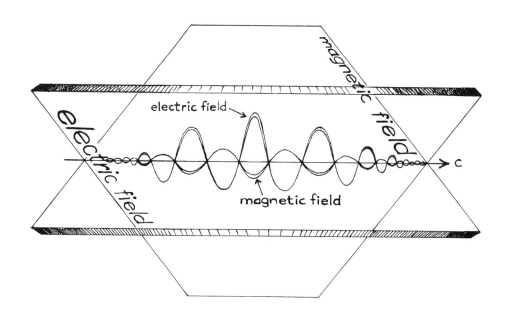

- X and γ rays are positioned on the electromagnetic spectrum with the highest energy, highest frequency, and shortest wavelengths.

- X and γ rays travel at the speed of light.

- The speed of light is 3×10^8 m/s ($c = 3 \times 10^8$ m/s).

- It is not possible to distinguish an x ray from a γ ray.

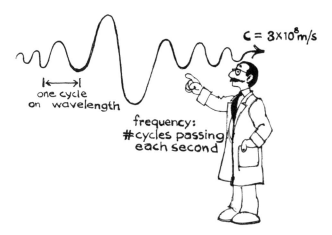

- The only difference between an x ray and a γ ray is origin. X rays come from the electron cloud; γ rays come from the nucleus.

$$1000eV = 10^3eV = 1keV$$

$$1000keV = 10^6eV = 1meV$$

- X and γ rays have no mass.

- The energy of an X or a γ ray is measured in electron volts (eV), kiloelectron volts (keV), or megaelectron volts (MeV).

- When x or γ rays interact with matter, they cause either electron excitation or ionization of an atom.

- Most x- and γ-ray interactions result in electronic excitation.

- The result of electronic excitation is heat and sometimes light.

- Ionization is the ejection of an electron from an atom.

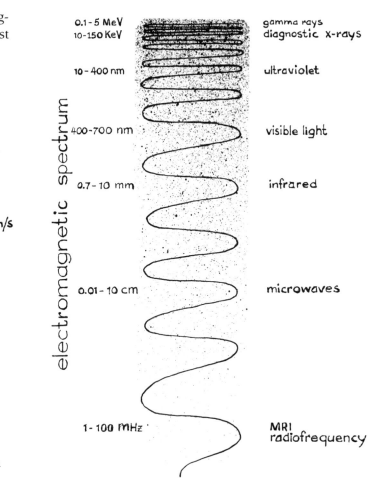

electromagnetic spectrum

0.1 - 5 MeV	gamma rays
10 - 150 KeV	diagnostic x-rays
10 - 400 nm	ultraviolet
400 - 700 nm	visible light
0.7 - 10 mm	infrared
0.01 - 10 cm	microwaves
1 - 100 MHz	MRI radiofrequency

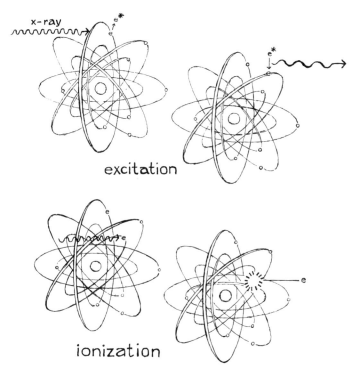

excitation

ionization

- The efficiency of a particular type of radiation in causing excitation and ionization is indicated by linear energy transfer (LET).

- LET has units of keV/μm, indicating energy deposited per unit path length.

- The LET of diagnostic x rays is 3.0 keV/μm.

- Ionization results in disruption of chemical and biochemical bonds in a molecule.

- Ionization forms the latent image in an x- or γ-ray image receptor.

- Ionization can have harmful biological effects on humans, such as cancer and leukemia.

Linear Energy Transfer

Radiation Therapy X-rays = 0.3 keV/μm

diagnostic x-rays = 3 keV/μm

beta particles = 3 keV/μm

alpha particles = 300 keV/μm

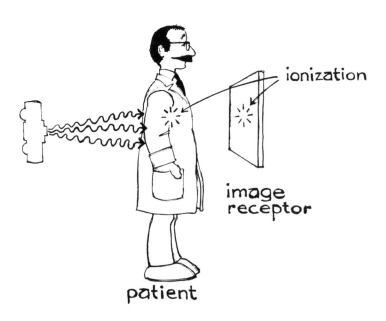

ionization

image receptor

patient

Chapter 2 Practice Questions

1. Mammography is a medical imaging procedure that employs
   a. nonionizing radiation.
   b. x rays.
   c. γ rays.
   d. ultrasound.

2. The radiation employed for diagnostic ultrasound is characterized by an approximate frequency range of
   a. 1 to 10 kHz.   c. 1 to 10 MHz.
   b. 1 to 100 kHz.   d. 1 to 100 MHz.

3. When used for medical imaging, γ rays are obtained
   a. by stopping high-speed electrons.
   b. by bending electrons in a magnetic field.
   c. from radioisotopes.
   d. from radio antennas.

4. The speed of light is
   a. 3×10^6 m/s.   c. 3×10^{10} m/s.
   b. 3×10^8 m/s.   d. 3×10^{12} m/s.

5. The fundamental unit of frequency is the
   a. electron volt (eV).   c. kilogram (kg).
   b. hertz (Hz).   d. joule (J).

6. The principal difference between x rays and γ rays is their
   a. energy.   c. mass.
   b. origin.   d. velocity.

7. The type of radiation employed for MRI can be characterized by its approximate frequency range of
   a. 1 to 10 kHz.   c. 1 to 10 MHz.
   b. 1 to 100 kHz.   d. 1 to 100 MHz.

8. Which of the following **is not** electromagnetic radiation?
   a. x rays   c. radio waves
   b. γ rays   d. ultrasound waves

9. X rays are produced
   a. in a radio antenna.
   b. with an oscillating surface.
   c. inside the nucleus of an atom.
   d. in the electron cloud of an atom.

10. Most x- and γ-ray interactions with tissue result in
    a. heat.   c. excitation.
    b. light.   d. ionization.

11. Nonionizing radiation is used in
    a. mammography.
    b. computed tomography.
    c. angiointerventional procedures.
    d. magnetic resonance imaging.

12. The source of diagnostic ultrasound is
    a. a vibrating surface.
    b. a radioisotope.
    c. a radio antenna.
    d. an electromagnetic wave.

13. Which of the following has the highest energy?

    a. x rays   c. microwaves
    b. visible light   d. radio frequencies

14. γ rays are produced

    a. in a radio antenna.
    b. with an oscillating surface.
    c. inside the nucleus of an atom.
    d. in the electron cloud of an atom.

15. The term **ionization** refers to

    a. adding particles.
    b. electromagnetic radiation.
    c. removal of an electron.
    d. disruption of a nucleus.

16. Diagnostic ultrasound employs

    a. nonionizing radiation.
    b. waveless radiation.
    c. photon-type radiation.
    d. radioactive material.

17. The source of energy used for magnetic resonance imaging is

    a. a vibrating surface.
    b. a radioisotope.
    c. a radio antenna.
    d. an electromagnetic wave.

18. Which of the following has the longest wavelength?

    a. x rays   c. microwaves
    b. visible light   d. radio frequencies

19. X and γ rays are usually identified according to their

    a. mass.   c. energy.
    b. velocity.   d. origin.

20. The latent image formed during x- or γ-ray imaging is the result of

    a. ionization.   c. crystallization.
    b. excitation.   d. polarization.

21. Medical imaging with radioisotopes uses

    a. nonionizing radiation.
    b. x rays.
    c. γ rays.
    d. radio frequencies.

22. When employed for medical imaging, x rays are obtained

    a. by stopping high-speed electrons.
    b. by bending electrons in a magnetic field.
    c. from radioisotopes.
    d. from radio antennas.

23. Which of the following has the highest frequency?

    a. x rays
    b. visible light
    c. microwaves
    d. radio frequencies

24. X- and γ-ray energy is measured in

    a. electron volt (eV).
    b. kilovolt peak (kVp).
    c. milliampere second (mAs).
    d. joule (J).

25. Human responses to x- or γ-ray exposure result principally from

    a. ionization.
    b. excitation.
    c. crystallization.
    d. polarization.

26. The speed of light is

    a. 3×10^6 cm/s.
    b. 3×10^8 cm/s.
    c. 3×10^{10} cm/s.
    d. 3×10^{12} cm/s.

27. Which of the following **does not** travel at the speed of light?

    a. x rays
    b. infrared radiation
    c. diagnostic ultrasound
    d. radio frequencies

28. The fundamental unit for measuring energy is the

    a. kilogram (kg).
    b. hertz (Hz).
    c. electron volt (eV).
    d. joule (J).

29. Electronic excitation is

    a. removal of an electron from an atom.
    b. polarization of an electron in an atom.
    c. raising an electron to a transient higher energy state.
    d. magnetically resonating an electron.

30. A mechanical wave in an elastic medium describes

    a. visible light.
    b. x rays.
    c. ultrasound.
    d. radio frequency.

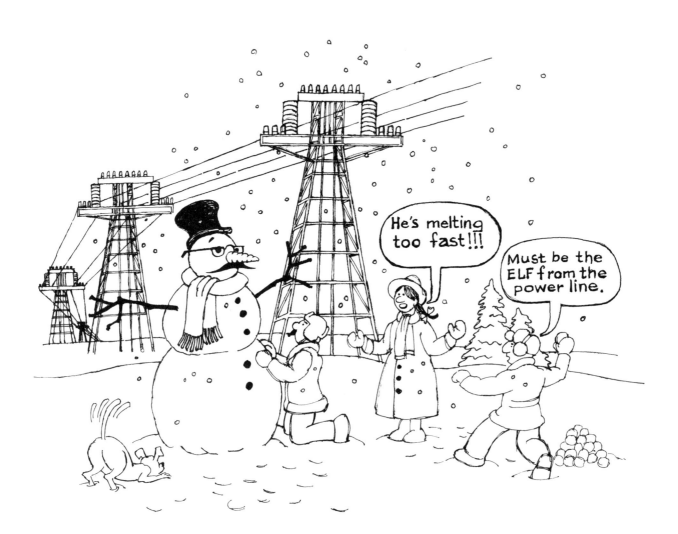

Measurement Units of Ionizing Radiation

- There are three units of radiation intensity and one unit of radioactivity.

- The classical units of radiation intensity are the roentgen (R), the radiation absorbed dose (rad), and the radiation equivalent man (rem).

- The international system (SI) of units of radiation intensity are the coulomb per kilogram (C/kg), the gray (Gy), and the sievert (Sv).

- The R and the C/kg are used to measure the intensity of x- and γ-ray ionization in air-termed **radiation exposure**.

- The coulomb is the unit of electrostatic charge. It is a measure of the number of electrons released in air by ionization.

Quantity	Classical Units	Standard International Units (SI)
exposure	roentgen (R)	coulomb/Kg
dose	rad	gray (Gy)
effective dose	rem	sievert (Sv)
radioactivity	curie (Ci)	becquerel (Bq)

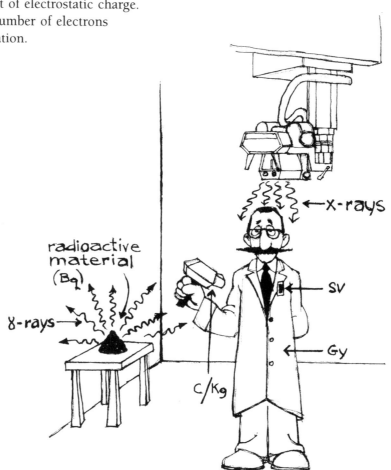

radioactive material (Bq)

←x-rays

Sv

Gy

γ-rays →

C/Kg

$$1R = 2.8 \times 10^{-4} \, C/Kg$$

$$1C = 1.6 \times 10^{19} \, electrons$$

$$1Kg = 2.2 \, lbs$$

$$1 \, rad = 100 \, erg/gm$$
$$1 \, Gy = 1 \, J/Kg$$
$$1 \, Gy = 100 \, rad$$

$$1 \, Sv = 100 \, rem$$

- The kilogram is the SI unit for mass. Multiply your weight in pounds by 0.455 to obtain your weight in kilograms.

- The rad and the gray are units of **radiation absorbed dose.**

- These units are used to express the amount of energy deposited in matter by ionizing radiation.

- Human responses to radiation are related to the magnitude of radiation absorbed dose.

- The erg, the electron volt (eV), and the joule (J) are units of energy.

- The fundamental unit of energy is the joule even though we measure x- and γ-ray energy in eV.

- The radiation unit employed for radiation protection purposes is either the rem or the sievert.

- The rem and the sievert are units of **effective dose.**

- The rem and the sievert take into account the type of radiation involved and the relative effect it has in causing a biological response.

- The type of radiation is signified by the radiation weighting factor W_R.

- W_R for x and γ rays used in medicine is equal to 1.

- For practical purposes, in medical imaging, 1 R = 1 rad = 1 rem.

- Units of radiation intensity cannot be used to express radioactivity.

Type of radiation	W_R
x - rays	1
γ - rays	1
electrons, positrons	1
neutrons	5 to 20 depending on energy
protons	2
alpha particles	20

- Radioactivity measures the quantity of radio-active material.

- Radioactivity refers to atoms having unstable nuclei that undergo spontaneous disintegration —radioactive decay—accompanied by the emission of ionizing radiation.

- Radioactivity is measured in curies (Ci) or becquerels (Bq).

$$1\,Ci = 3.7 \times 10^{10}\,d/s$$
atoms disintegrating per second
$$1\,Bq = 1\,d/s$$
$$1\,Ci = 3.7 \times 10^{10}\,Bq$$

Chapter 3 Practice Questions

1. Which of the following is the unit of radiation exposure?
   a. gray (Gy)
   b. rem
   c. coulombs per kilogram (C/kg)
   d. joule (J)

2. Which of the following is an SI unit?
   a. rad
   b. roentgen (R)
   c. becquerel (Bq)
   d. curie (Ci)

3. One rad is equal to
   a. 100 erg/g.
   b. 100 erg/kg.
   c. 1 J/kg.
   d. 100 Gy.

4. The radiation weighting factor W_R is used to convert
   a. effective dose to dose.
   b. exposure to dose.
   c. exposure to effective dose.
   d. dose to effective dose.

5. One becquerel (Bq) is equal to
   a. 1 d/s.
   b. 100 d/s.
   c. 2.2×10^{10} d/s.
   d. 3.7×10^{10} d/s.

6. Which of the following is a unit of radiation dose?
   a. gray (Gy)
   b. joule (J)
   c. roentgen (R)
   d. curie (Ci)

7. A unit of radiation exposure is one that measures
   a. ionization in air.
   b. energy deposited in tissue.
   c. occupational exposure.
   d. radioactivity.

8. One gray is equal to
   a. 100 erg/g.   c. 1 J/g.
   b. 100 erg/kg.   d. 1 J/kg.

9. The radiation weighting factor W_R distinguishes among different types of radiation according to their
   a. energy.
   b. linear energy transfer (LET).
   c. intensity.
   d. velocity.

10. Ten millicuries of ^{99m}Tc is equivalent to
    a. 3.7 Bq.   c. 37 MBq.
    b. 3.7 mBq.   d. 370 GBq.

11. Which of the following is most important in assessing human radiation responses?
    a. radiation absorbed dose
    b. radiation exposure
    c. linear energy transfer
    d. effective dose

12. Which of the following is a unit of effective dose?
    a. roentgen (R)   c. joule (J)
    b. sievert (Sv)   d. becquerel (Bq)

13. What unit is a measure of a quantity of electrons?
    a. joule (J)   c. roentgen (R)
    b. coulomb (C)   d. hertz (Hz)

14. Units of radiation dose measure
    a. ionization in air.
    b. energy deposited in tissue.
    c. radioactivity.
    d. occupational exposure.

15. The value for the radiation weighting factor W_R for x and γ rays used in medical imaging is
    a. 1.   c. 10.
    b. 5.   d. 20.

16. If the precautionary limit placed on radon gas by the U.S. Environmental Protection Agency (USEPA) were 1 pCi/l, it would be equal to
    a. 0.037 Bq/l.   c. 370 Bq/l.
    b. 3.7 Bq/l.   d. 37 kBq/l.

17. The LET of diagnostic x-rays is closest to
    a. 0.1 keV/μm.   c. 1.0 keV/μm.
    b. 0.3 keV/μm.   d. 3.0 keV/μm.

18. Which of the following is a unit of radioactivity?

    a. joule (J)   c. rem
    b. becquerel (Bq)   d. gray (Gy)

19. The SI unit for mass is the

    a. pound (lb).   c. kilogram (kg).
    b. gram (g).   d. joule (J).

20. Which of the following **is not** a unit of energy?

    a. erg   c. joule
    b. coulomb   d. electron volt

21. The SI unit of radioactivity is the

    a. curie (Ci).   c. joule (J).
    b. becquerel (Bq).   d. kilogram (kg).

22. How many millicuries are there in 1 Ci?

    a. 10   c. 1,000
    b. 100   d. 1,000,000

23. Which of the following **is not** an SI unit?

    a. roentgen (R)   c. sievert (Sv)
    b. gray (Gy)   d. becquerel (Bq)

24. An imaging technologist weighs 110 lb. What is her approximate mass in kilograms?

    a. 10 kg   c. 50 kg
    b. 30 kg   d. 70 kg

25. Which of the following is employed for radiation protection purposes?

    a. radiation exposure
    b. radiation dose
    c. radiation dose equivalent
    d. radioactivity

26. One curie is equal to

    a. 3.7×10^{10} d/s.   c. 2.2×10^{10} d/s.
    b. 3.7×10^{12} d/s.   d. 2.2×10^{12} d/s.

27. How many becquerels (Bq) are there in one megabecquerel (MBq)?

    a. 10 (10^1)   c. 1,000 (10^3)
    b. 100 (10^2)   d. 1,000,000 (10^6)

28. The precautionary limit placed on radon gas by the USEPA is

    a. 1 pCi/l.   c. 4 pCi/l.
    b. 2 pCi/l.   d. 8 pCi/l.

29. The standard person defined for radiation protection purposes has a mass of 70 kg. What is his weight in pounds?

    a. 77 lb   c. 154 lb
    b. 105 lb   d. 202 lb

30. How many becquerels (Bq) are there in one gigabecquerel (Gbq)?
    - a. 10^3
    - b. 10^6
    - c. 10^9
    - d. 10^{12}

31. One curie is equal to
    - a. 3.7×10^{10} d/min.
    - b. 3.7×10^{12} d/min.
    - c. 2.2×10^{10} d/min.
    - d. 2.2×10^{12} d/min.

32. Radiation absorbed dose is principally related to
    - a. ionization per unit path length in air.
    - b. ionization per unit path length in tissue.
    - c. energy deposited per unit path length in tissue.
    - d. energy deposited per unit mass of tissue.

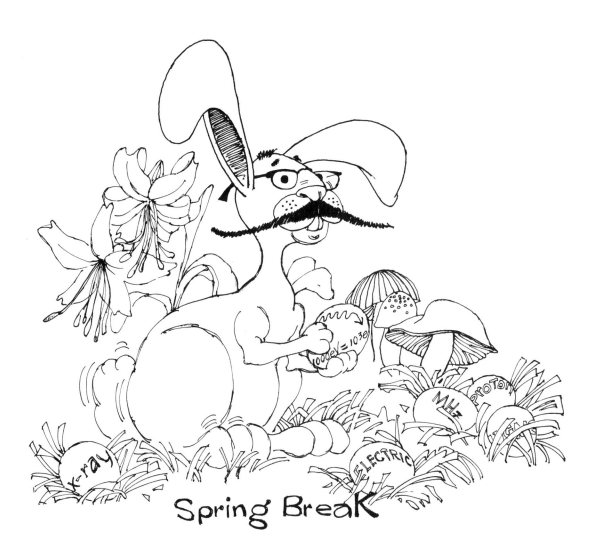

Sources of Ionizing Radiation

- All ionizing radiation can be classified according to whether it is manmade or occurs naturally.

- The largest source of manmade radiation is from **x-ray imaging**, which averages 40 mrem/y to the U.S. population.

- The second largest source of manmade radiation is from **nuclear medicine procedures**, resulting in a dose of approximately 14 mrem/y to the U.S. population.

- Minor sources of manmade radiation are nuclear power plants, consumer products, and research applications. These activities result in an average dose of 10 mrem/y to the U.S. population.

- In the United States, the total annual dose from manmade radiation is estimated to be 65 mrem.

- There are three sources of naturally occurring radiation to which the entire body is exposed.

- One additional source affects only the lung.

Manmade Ionizing Radiation

Diagnostic x-rays:	39 mrem/y
Nuclear Medicine :	14 mrem/y
Consumer products:	10 mrem/y
Other :	2 mrem/y
Total	**65** mrem/y

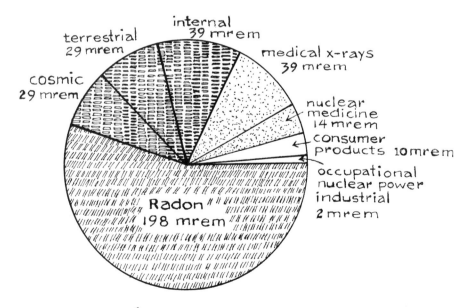

Total 360 mrem

23

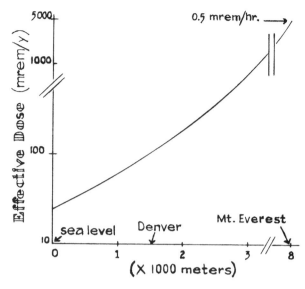

Cosmic Radiation

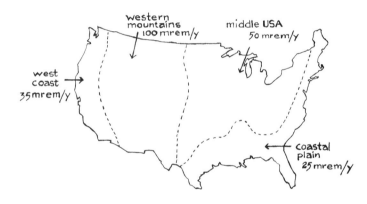

Terrestrial Radiation

Terrestrial Radiation Sources

potassium - 40	^{40}K	$1.3 \times 10^9 y$
rubidium - 87	^{87}Rb	$5 \times 10^{10} y$
thorium - 232	^{232}Th	$1.4 \times 10^{10} y$
uranium - 238	^{238}U	$4.5 \times 10^9 y$

- **Cosmic radiation** contributes approximately 30 mrem/y.

- Cosmic radiation increases with latitude because charged particle radiation, such as solar flare protons, are redirected by the earth's magnetic field.

- Cosmic radiation intensity is lowest at the equator and highest at the poles.

- Cosmic radiation intensity increases with altitude because at higher altitudes there is less atmosphere to serve as an absorber.

- The cosmic ray intensity at Houston, Texas (elevation 10 m), is approximately 25 mrem/y, while that at the summit of Mount Everest (elevation 8,848 m) is approximately 4,000 mrem/y or 0.5 mrem/h.

- **Terrestrial radiation** results from radioisotopes in the earth.

- Terrestrial radioisotopes were created at the time of the earth's formation, approximately 4.5×10^9 years ago, and therefore have equally long half-lives.

- The principal radioisotopes that contribute to terrestrial radiation are potassium-40, thorium-232, and uranium-238 and daughters.

- Terrestrial radiation varies widely throughout the United States and depends on the composition of the earth at any given location.

- In the United States exposure from terrestrial radiation is 29 mrem/y.

- Terrestrial radiation exposure levels range from a low of approximately 25 mrem/y along the Texas Gulf Coast to a high of 100 mrem/y on the Colorado plateau.

- Throughout life we are continuously exposed to very small **internal sources of radiation**.

- Naturally occurring radioisotopes in body tissues contribute 39 mrem/y to our total radiation dose.

- The principal sources of internal radiation are potassium-40, carbon-14, and decay products of polonium-210.

- Moving to another location can reduce exposure to cosmic radiation and to terrestrial radiation, but nothing can be done to reduce internal radiation exposure.

- **Lung tissue** is exposed to radiation emitted by radon-222 (^{222}Rn).

- ^{222}Rn is a naturally occurring gas whose concentration in the atmosphere depends on many factors, mainly the underlying earth.

- ^{222}Rn results from the radioactive decay of radium-226 (^{226}Ra).

- ^{222}Rn adheres to dust particles in the air, which are breathed in and lodge in the alveolar spaces of the lung.

- ^{222}Rn has a short half-life (2.3 days), but it emits α particles which have $W_R = 20$.

- The average annual dose to the lung from ^{222}Rn in the United States is 200 mrem/y.

- There is a considerable variation in radon intensity throughout the United States.

- The USEPA recommends corrective action when radon levels exceed 4 pCi/l in a home or office.

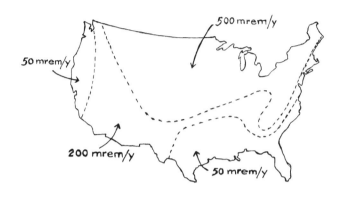

Internal Radiation Sources

potassium - 40	^{40}K	17 mrem/y
carbon - 14	^{14}C	10 mrem/y
polonium - 210	^{210}Po -	
To lead - 210	^{210}Pb	12 mrem/y
Total		**39 mrem/y**

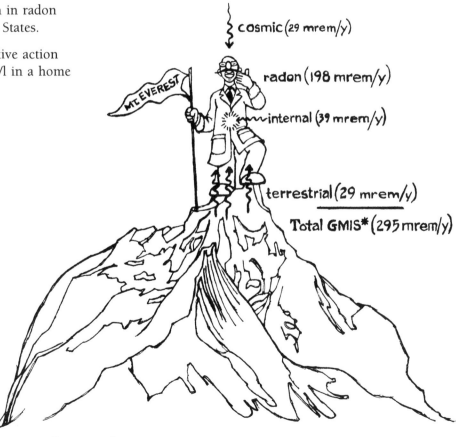

Radon Exposure

cosmic (29 mrem/y)

radon (198 mrem/y)

internal (39 mrem/y)

terrestrial (29 mrem/y)

Total GMIS* (295 mrem/y)

MT EVEREST

* God Made It So

Chapter 4 Practice Questions

1. Which of the following contributes the highest radiation dose to humans?
   a. medical imaging   c. cosmic radiation
   b. manmade radiation   d. radon

2. Which of the following sources of natural radiation exposure **does not** vary with location?
   a. radon
   b. terrestrial radiation
   c. internally deposited radionuclides
   d. cosmic radiation

3. In the United States the average exposure from terrestrial radiation sources is approximately
   a. 10 mrem/y.   c. 30 mrem/y.
   b. 20 mrem/y.   d. 50 mrem/y.

4. Radon gas is created
   a. because of the earth's magnetic field.
   b. because of the earth's rotation.
   c. by radioactive decay of ^{14}C.
   d. by radioactive decay of ^{226}Ra.

5. The average dose to Americans from medical x-ray imaging is approximately
   a. 20 mrem/y.   c. 54 mrem/y.
   b. 40 mrem/y.   d. 65 mrem/y.

6. Cosmic radiation intensity
   a. decreases with increasing altitude.
   b. decreases with increasing latitude.
   c. is highest at the poles.
   d. is highest at the equator.

7. The approximate radiation exposure from cosmic radiation in the United States is
   a. 10 mrem/y.   c. 30 mrem/y.
   b. 20 mrem/y.   d. 50 mrem/y.

8. At any given location, the radon concentration
   a. varies considerably.
   b. is constant from day to day.
   c. is constant from month to month.
   d. is constant seasonally.

9. The average dose to Americans from all medical imaging procedures is approximately
   a. 20 mrem/y.   c. 54 mrem/y.
   b. 40 mrem/y.   d. 65 mrem/y.

10. Terrestrial radiation exposure depends principally on
    a. radionuclides deposited in the earth.
    b. latitude.
    c. altitude.
    d. the earth's magnetic field.

11. The approximate radiation exposure from internally deposited radionuclides is
    a. 10 mrem/y.   c. 30 mrem/y.
    b. 20 mrem/y.   d. 50 mrem/y.

12. The average dose to Americans from all sources of manmade radiation is approximately
    a. 20 mrem/y.   c. 54 mrem/y.
    b. 40 mrem/y.   d. 65 mrem/y.

13. Which of the following radionuclides is a principal constituent of terrestrial radiation sources?
    a. ^{226}Ra   c. ^{14}C
    b. ^{40}K   d. ^{131}I

14. The annual radiation dose to the lung from radon gas is estimated to be
    a. 50 mrem.   c. 200 mrem.
    b. 100 mrem.   d. 250 mrem.

15. Which of the following **does not** contribute to the whole-body radiation dose?
    a. radon
    b. terrestrial radiation
    c. cosmic radiation
    d. internally deposited radionuclides

16. Which of the following is a principal internally deposited radionuclide?
    a. ^{226}Ra   c. ^{238}U
    b. ^{40}K   d. ^{131}I

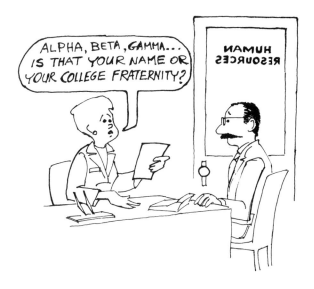

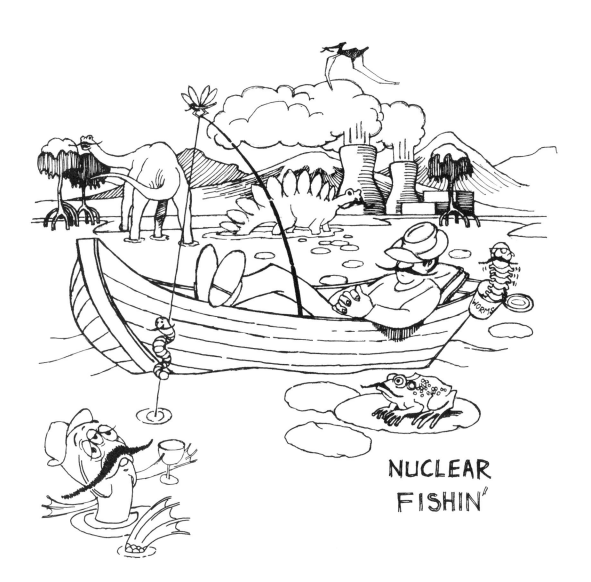

NUCLEAR FISHIN'

Biological Effects of Ionizing Radiation

- Although radiation interaction occurs with electrons, the result is a chain reaction—involving the disruption of molecular bonds, an alteration in biochemical pathways, transformation of a cell, and observable effects at the tissue or whole-body level.

- The ability of a particular type of radiation to produce a response is called its **relative biological effectiveness (RBE)**.

- The RBE of diagnostic x rays equals 1.0.

AT THE MOLECULAR LEVEL

- Most interactions between radiation and tissue occur with water because water is the most abundant molecule in the body.

- If interaction with water were only electron excitation, the only response would be temperature elevation.

- When water is ionized by radiation, free radicals are formed.

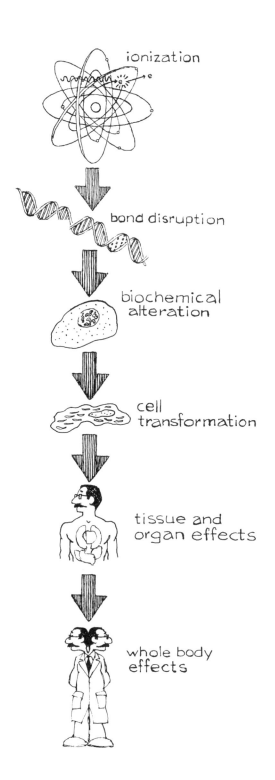

29

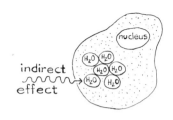

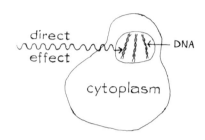

$$\left(H_2O\right) + \rightsquigarrow \rightarrow \left(HOH\right)^+ + e^-$$

$$\left(H_2O\right) + e^- \rightarrow \left(HOH\right)^-$$

$$\left(HOH\right)^+ \rightarrow H^+ + \left(OH^*\right)$$

$$\left(HOH\right)^- \rightarrow OH^- + \left(H^*\right)$$

* = free radicals

Atoms of the Body

60% hydrogen
25.7% oxygen
10.7% carbon
2.4% nitrogen
0.2% calcium
0.1% phosphorus
0.1% sulphur
0.8% trace elements

Molecules of the body

80% water
15% protein
2% lipids
1% carbohydrates
1% nucleic acid
1% other

- Radiation interaction at the molecular level is either via a direct effect or an indirect effect.

- When interaction is via a direct effect, it occurs in an atom of the **target molecule**.

- Target molecules are few in number but are exceptionally important to the cell.

- In both genetic and somatic cells, the target molecule is deoxyribonucleic acid (DNA).

- Very few molecular changes occur via a direct effect because DNA is a rare molecule.

- When radiation interacts via an indirect effect, free radicals are formed.

- **Free radicals** are molecules with excess energy that diffuse through the cell and disrupt molecular bonds of target molecules.

- Free radicals exist for less than 1 ms.

- Free radicals are produced principally from the interaction of radiation with water.

- Water is the most abundant molecule in the body—approximately 60% of all molecules are water.

- Free radicals are more easily produced in the presence of oxygen. Most tissues are oxygenated, which enhances free radical production.

- An indirect effect can also occur by radiation interaction with the three most abundant macromolecules—lipids, carbohydrates, and proteins.

AT THE CELLULAR LEVEL

- Every human cell has two main parts: cytoplasm and a nucleus.

- The cytoplasm is very radiation-resistant; when only the cytoplasm is irradiated, approximately 1,000 rad is necessary to produce cell death.

- The cytoplasm is radiation-resistant because the target molecule DNA is not in the cytoplasm.

- The target molecule DNA is in the nucleus, and therefore the nucleus is very radiosensitive.

- When the nucleus is irradiated, only approximately 100 rads is required to kill a cell.

- Radiation-induced cell death is represented by single-cell survival curves, of which there are two basic kinds.

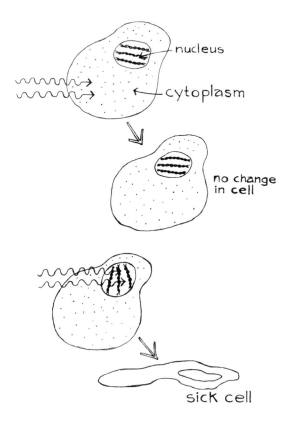

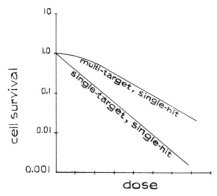

- These cell survival curves are always plotted on semilog paper in order to accommodate the enormous range of cells necessary for the study.

- If radiation interacted with cells uniformly, there would be a dose, say 100 rad, that could kill all cells.

- Radiation interaction with cells via either a direct or an indirect effect is random; therefore some cells always escape death.

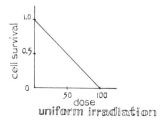

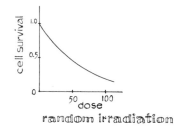

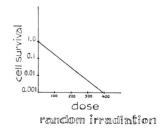

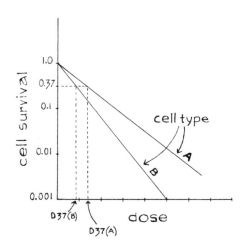

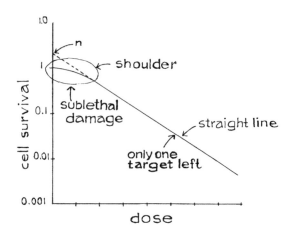

- Primitive cells like virus particles and bacteria follow the single-target, single-hit dose-response relationship.

- When irradiated with high-LET radiation such as α particles, human cells follow the single-target, single-hit dose-response relationship.

- The extrapolation number or target number (n) for the single-target, single-hit dose-response relationship is 1.

- For the single-target, single-hit model, the value of D_{37} indicates the relative radio-sensitivity of that type of cell.

- The parameter D_{37} is the dose that would kill all cells if delivered uniformly.

- Since radiation interacts randomly, D_{37} is the dose that kills 63% of the cells, allowing 37% to survive.

- Thirty-seven percent of the cells survive because 37% of the radiation is wasted on targets hit more than once.

- The mathematics of cell survival following the random interaction of radiation obey Poisson's law of statistics.

- The model of cell killing for human cells is the multitarget, single-hit dose-response relationship.

- According to the multitarget, single-hit dose-response relationship, human cells must accumulate **sublethal damage** because human cells have more than one sensitive target.

- Sublethal damage is represented by the shoulder of the multitarget, single-hit dose-response relationship.

- Once beyond the shoulder of the multitarget, single-hit dose-response relationship, human cells exhibit a single-target, single-hit response to radiation.

- Once beyond the shoulder of the multitarget, single-hit dose-response relationship, all targets in each cell except one have been hit and inactivated.

- When the straight-line region of the multi-target, single-hit model is extrapolated to the y axis, the intersection is the value of the extrapolation number or target number n.

- Human cells have target numbers ranging from approximately 2 to 10.

- In the straight-line portion of the multitarget, single-hit dose-response relationship, the dose that can reduce the surviving fraction to 37% is called the **mean lethal dose** (D_0).

- D_0 is the dose that, in the straight-line region, would have killed 100% of the remaining cells if it had been delivered **uniformly**.

- D_0 results in 37% survival for cells in the straight-line region of the multitarget, single-hit dose-response relationship.

- Generally, the larger D_0, the more resistant the cells are to radiation.

- The larger the target number n, the more targets there are in the cell, each of which has to be hit in order for the cell to die.

- The larger the target number n, the more resistant the cells are to radiation.

- The shoulder dose D_Q measures the width of the shoulder of the multitarget, single-hit dose-response relationship.

- D_Q is a measure of the amount of **sublethal damage** that a cell can sustain.

- The value of D_Q is obtained by dropping a line to the dose axis from the intersection of the line representing 100% survival and the line representing extrapolation of the linear portion of the curve.

- The larger D_Q, the more resistant to radiation are the cells.

- The mean lethal dose D_0, the target number n, and the shoulder dose D_Q are three measures of radiosensitivity for a particular type of cell.

- When only one parameter is employed to express cell sensitivity to radiation, it is D_0.

- If the same cells are irradiated with low-LET radiation, D_0 is higher.

- If the same cells are irradiated with less oxygen present, D_0 is higher.

- If the same cells are irradiated with either dose fractionation or dose protraction, D_0 is higher.

- The term **transformation** refers to changing a normal cell into a malignant cell.

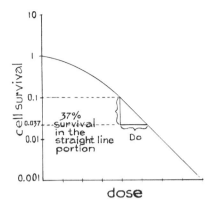

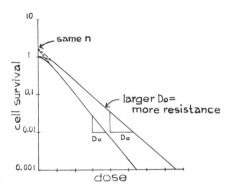

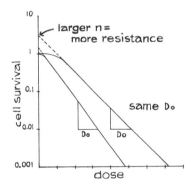

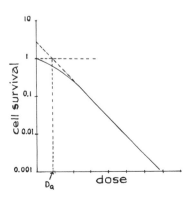

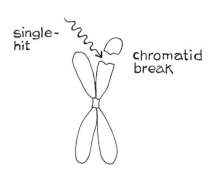

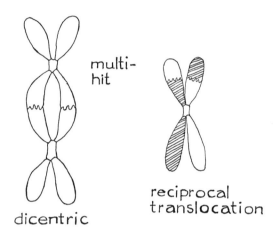

Tissue Radiosensitivity

high: lymphoid tissue
bone marrow
gonads

intermediate: skin
G I Tract
Kidney

low: muscle
brain
spine

- Chromosomal aberrations are a good indication of radiation exposure.

- There are two types of chromosomal aberrations—single-hit and multihit.

- Chromosome deletions and chromatid breaks are single-hit aberrations.

- Dicentrics, multicentrics, and ring chromosomes are multihit aberrations.

- Reciprocal translocation is one type of multihit aberration that requires a karyotype for detection.

- **Karyotyping** is the process of aligning the 44 somatic chromosomes in pairs according to size and positioning the two sex chromosomes separately.

AT THE TISSUE AND ORGAN LEVELS

- Radiation damage to a cell can result in injury to tissues and organs if the radiation dose is very high. The principal effect is **atrophy** or reduction in size.

- The most radiation-sensitive tissues are lymphoid and hematological.

- The most radiation-resistant tissues are bone and nervous tissue.

- The most radiation-sensitive organs are the small intestines and kidneys.

- The most radiation-resistant organs are the brain and heart.

- These classifications of radiation sensitivity apply only to high-dose effects, which are not normally experienced in diagnostic imaging.

AT THE WHOLE-BODY LEVEL

- Human responses to radiation exposure are classified as either early effects or late effects.

- **Early effects** occur within weeks or months of a high dose of radiation—one exceeding 25 rad.

- Early effects are termed **deterministic** effects—the severity of the effect is dose-related.

- The lethal dose to 50% of a population dying within 60 days of exposure is termed **LD**$_{50/60}$.

- The **LD**$_{50/60}$ for humans is approximately 350 rad.

- Skin erythema and moist desquamation are early effects.

- Following chronic irradiation the threshold dose required to produce erythema is approximately 600 rad, and that for moist desquamation is several thousand rad.

- Tissue atrophy, shrinkage, is an early effect, and approximately 1,000 rad is necessary to produce this effect.

- Tissue atrophy is a planned, deliberate part of radiation oncology.

- Changes in the peripheral blood, hematological changes, are early effects of radiation exposure.

- Every type of peripheral blood cell is reduced in number following radiation exposure.

- Among the blood cells lymphocytes are the most sensitive to radiation exposure. Responses to a dose as low as 10 rad can be measured.

- The effect on the testes is an early effect.

- A 10-rad testicular dose results in a measurable reduction in sperm count.

- Chromosomal aberrations can be either early effects or late effects.

- As time following radiation exposure lengthens, the ratio of multihit to single-hit aberrations increases.

- Chromosomal aberrations are scored during the metaphase portion of mitosis.

- Most early effects of radiation exposure are of no concern in medical imaging, where radiation doses are very low. The one exception is skin damage in patients undergoing various angiointerventional procedures.

- **Late effects** of radiation exposure occur years after exposure to low doses of radiation, less than 25 rad.

- Late effects are termed **stochastic effects**—the incidence of response is dose-related.

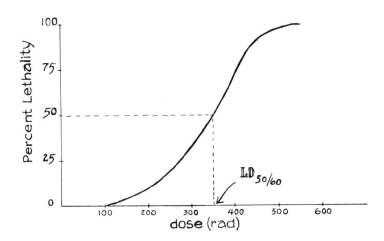

Early Radiation Effect	Minimum Dose	Risk
reproductive response	10 rad	sterility = 500 rad
chromosome aberration	10 rad	
skin erythema	200 rad	SED$_{50}$ = 600 rad
low blood count	25 rad	
death	100 rad	LD$_{50/60}$ = 350 rad

Early Effects – deterministic, dose threshold, severity proportional to dose

Late Effects – stochastic, no dose threshold, incidence proportional to dose

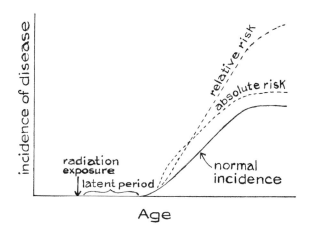

The Percent of Americans
who will die of :

heart disease – 56%
cancer   – 21%
stroke   – 5%
accidents   – 3%
firearms   – 2%
radiation   – ?

- The risk of a stochastic effect is measured as either a relative or an absolute factor.

- Relative risk is the ratio of observed incidence to expected incidence and is usually expressed as a ratio.

- Absolute risk is the additional cases of disease in an exposed population and is usually expressed as number of cases per 100,000/y/rad.

- Premature aging resulting in life shortening is a late effect estimated at 10 days of life lost per rad.

- Premature aging and life-span shortening are of no concern to medical imaging personnel.

- Some radiation effects on local tissue are of concern in medical imaging.

- Radiation exposure can cause cataracts in the lens of the eye.

- Radiation-induced cataracts are distinct from naturally occurring cataracts in that they form on the posterior pole of the lens.

- Radiation-induced cataracts exhibit a threshold dose of x- or γ-ray exposure of approximately 200 rad acute exposure or 1,000 rad chronic exposure.

- Radiation-induced cataracts are of little concern in medical imaging.

- Irradiation of the gonads is a local tissue late effect of some concern in diagnostic imaging.

- The principal concern is for patients rather than personnel.

- An acute dose of approximately 200 rad may produce transient infertility; 500 rad is required for sterility.

- No harmful effect of gonadal irradiation has ever been observed in radiology personnel.

- No harmful effect has been observed in patients; still the potential for harm is there, and consequently gonadal shields are recommended.

- Radiation-induced **malignant disease** is the principal health hazard of medical imaging.

- Approximately 20% of Americans die of cancer, making radiation-induced cancer very hard to detect.

- Bone cancer has been observed in radium watch dial painters.

- Approximately 10% of all females will develop breast cancer.

- Breast cancer has been observed in fluoroscopically treated tuberculosis (TB) patients, in patients receiving radiotherapy for postpartum mastitis, and in atomic bomb survivors.

- Thyroid cancer has been observed in children irradiated for thymus enlargement as newborns, in children on South Sea islands during nuclear weapons testing, and in Israeli children whose scalps were irradiated to control ringworm.

- Thyroid cancer has not been observed in populations exposed to diagnostic levels of ^{131}I.

- Excess radiation-induced lung cancer has been observed in uranium miners, in atomic bomb survivors, and in patients treated with x-ray therapy for ankylosing spondylitis.

- Liver cancer has been observed in early angiography patients where the contrast medium was radioactive thorium dioxide.

- Leukemia has been observed in patients treated with radiation for ankylosing spondylitis, in women treated with radiation for cervical cancer, and in atomic bomb survivors.

- The minimum latent period for radiation-induced leukemia is 2 to 3 years.

- The risk of developing cancer and leukemia induced by radiation is 1×10^{-4} rem^{-1}. This risk coefficient for cancer and leukemia is obtained from analysis of human radiation exposure.

- Because there is no dose threshold for radiation-induced malignant disease, we recommend radiation exposure be maintained as low as reasonably achievable (ALARA) in all areas of medical imaging.

- Maintain patient and personnel exposure as low as reasonably achievable.

- Exposure of pregnant women to radiation is of considerable concern in diagnostic imaging.

Radiation induced cancer in humans

Population	Cancer
radium watch dial painters	bone cancer
Fluoroscopically Treated TB Patients	breast cancer
Childhood irradiation for thymic enlargement	thyroid cancer
uranium miners	lung cancer
Thorotrast patients	liver cancer
Ankylosing Spondylitis patients	leukemia
A-bomb survivors	leukemia breast cancer

- The first 2 weeks of pregnancy are the safest because the only response is resorption of the conceptus and therefore no pregnancy.

- During the second to tenth weeks of pregnancy, the most likely response is a congenital abnormality.

- During any stage of pregnancy, radiation can induce a malignancy that will appear during childhood.

- The first trimester is more sensitive than the second trimester which is more sensitive than the third trimester.

Effect of a 10-rad Fetal dose

Time of exposure	Type of response	Natural Occurrence	Radiation Response
0-2 weeks	Spontaneous abortion	25%	0.1%
2-10 weeks	Congenital abnormalities	5%	1%
2-15 weeks	Mental retardation	6%	0.5%
0-9 months	Malignant disease	8/10,000	12/10,000
0-9 months	Impaired growth & development	1%	nil
0-9 months	Genetic mutations	10%	nil

Chapter 5 Practice Questions

1. The chain of events following radiation exposure proceeds from
   a. bond disruption to biochemical alteration to cellular transformation to whole-body effects.
   b. bond disruption to cellular transformation to biochemical alteration to whole-body effects.
   c. biochemical alteration to bond disruption to cellular transformation to whole-body effects.
   d. biochemical alteration to cellular transformation to bond disruption to whole-body effects.

2. Most radiation interaction with tissue occurs with
   a. water.   c. proteins.
   b. carbohydrates. d. nucleic acids.

3. Which of the following human responses to radiation exposure is classified as an early effect?
   a. breast cancer
   b. leukemia
   c. chromosomal aberrations
   d. cataracts

4. When tissue is oxygenated,

   a. a higher dose is required for a given effect.
   b. DNA becomes radiation-resistant.
   c. cell death is less likely.
   d. more free radicals are formed.

5. Radiation-induced cancer usually exhibits a latent period of

   a. less than 1 year.
   b. 1 to 3 years.
   c. 3 to 10 years.
   d. more than 10 years.

6. Hematological changes following radiation exposure refer to

   a. injury to skin.
   b. reduction in peripheral blood cells.
   c. loss of hair.
   d. cataracts.

7. Approximately how many of us are likely to die of cancer?

   a. 5%   c. 20%
   b. 10%   d. 40%

8. Because radiation interaction is random, a dose equal to D_{37} is expected to kill what percentage of cells?

   a. 0   c. 63
   b 37   d. 100

9. An early effect of radiation exposure on humans that is of current concern in medical x-ray imaging is

   a. chromosomal aberrations.
   b. cataracts.
   c. epilation (loss of hair).
   d. skin erythema.

10. Which of the following is considered a late radiation response?

    a. sterility
    b. lung cancer
    c. skin erythema
    d. hematological depression

11. The RBE of diagnostic x rays has a value of

    a. 0.1.   c. 1.0.
    b. 0.5.   d. 5.0.

12. In general, when evaluating cellular radiosensitivity,

    a. cells with a large D_0 are more sensitive.
    b. cells with higher target numbers are more sensitive.
    c. cells with a smaller D_Q are more sensitive.
    d. anoxic cells are more sensitive.

13. The principal target molecules in the body are

    a. water.   c. proteins.
    b. carbohydrates.   d. DNA.

14. Which of the following **is not** a macromolecule?

    a. lipid

    b. carbohydrate

    c. protein

    d. water

15. Radiation-induced chromosomal aberrations are scored during which phase of the cell cycle?

    a. G1   c. G2

    b. S   d. M

16. What dose-response relationship describes the effect of radiation on bacteria?

    a. single-target, single-hit

    b. single-target, multihit

    c. multitarget, single-hit

    d. multitarget, multihit

17. Which of the following populations have experienced an excessive incidence of breast cancer?

    1. atomic bomb survivors

    2. postpartum mastitis cardiotherapy patients

    3. TB patients who have undergone fluoroscopy

    4. patients in a large-scale mammography screening

    a. Only 1, 2, and 3 are correct.

    b. Only 1 and 3 are correct.

    c. Only 2 and 4 are correct.

    d. All are correct.

18. In this example of a multitarget, single-hit model of cell survival, which region represents the mean lethal dose?

    a. A   c. C

    b. B   d. D

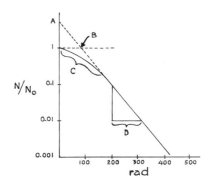

19. The principal health hazard for patients and medical x-ray workers is

    a. malignant disease.

    b. cataracts.

    c. congenital abnormalities.

    d. life-span shortening.

20. The target molecule is defined as one
    a. with which radiation interacts.
    b. that produces free radicals.
    c. that has a chainlike form and can be broken.
    d. that is low in number but critical to cell function.

21. Which of the following is most abundant in the human body?
    a. DNA   c. carbohydrates
    b. lipids   d. proteins

22. When only the cytoplasm is irradiated, the dose required to kill a cell is approximately
    a. 10 rad.   c. 1,000 rad.
    b. 100 rad.   d. 10,000 rad.

23. Radiation-induced leukemia usually follows a latent period of
    a. less than 2 years.   c. 6 to 12 years.
    b. 2 to 6 years.   d. more than 12 years.

24. Radiation-induced chromosome aberrations are scored during which phase of the cell cycle?
    a. prophase   c. anaphase
    b. metaphase   d. telophase

25. The mathematics on which cell survival radiation dose-response relationships are based are described by
    a. Roentgen.   c. Coulomb.
    b. Poisson.   d. Hertz.

26. During which period of pregnancy is irradiation of the embryo or fetus safest?
    a. the first 2 weeks
    b. weeks 3 through 10
    c. the second trimester
    d. the third trimester

27. Which of the following is not a somatic cell?
    a. red blood cell   c. oocyte
    b. neuron   d. connective tissue

28. The two principal parts of every human cell are
    a. membrane and cytoplasm.
    b. cytoplasm and nucleus.
    c. nucleus and lysosome.
    d. lysosome and membrane.

29. Human responses to radiation exposure that are late effects
    a. occur within weeks or months.
    b. required a dose exceeding 25 rad.
    c. are called deterministic.
    d. are called stochastic.

30. Which dose-response relationship describes the irradiation of human cells with high-LET radiation?
    a. single-target, single-hit
    b. single-target, multihit
    c. multitarget, single-hit
    d. multitarget, multihit

31. In the linear portion of the multitarget, single-hit radiation dose-response relationship
    a. no critical targets have yet been hit.
    b. one critical target in each cell has been hit.
    c. all but one critical target in each cell have been hit.
    d. all critical targets in each cell have been hit.

32. In general, when evaluating cellular radiosensitivity,
    a. cells with a small D_0 are more sensitive.
    b. cells with higher target numbers are more sensitive.
    c. cells with a higher D_0 are more sensitive.
    d. anoxic cells are more sensitive.

33. Which of the following describes a deterministic effect of radiation?
    a. incidence increasing with increasing dose
    b. severity increasing with increasing dose
    c. an effect following an acute dose
    d. an effect following a chronic dose

34. Most interactions between radiation and tissue occur via
    a. a direct effect.   c. somatic radicals.
    b. an indirect effect.   d. genetic cells.

35. When evaluating cell radiosensitivity,
    a. more free radicals are formed in the nucleus than in the cytoplasm.
    b. the cytoplasm contains the target molecules.
    c. the cytoplasm is more radiation-resistant than the nucleus.
    d. the nucleus is protected by a membrane.

36. A stochastic effect of radiation exposure
    a. refers to molecular effects.
    b. requires free radical production.
    c. occurs when the incidence of response is dose-dependent.
    d. occurs when the severity of response is dose-dependent.

37. In this example of a multitarget, single-hit radiation dose-response relationship, which represents the accumulation of sublethal damage?

    a. A   c. C
    b. B   d. D

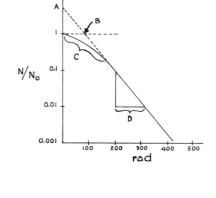

38. Human cells have target numbers ranging from

    a. 0 to 1.   c. 1 to 5.
    b. 1 to 2.   d. 2 to 10.

39. Which of the following tissues is most radiation-resistant?

    a. nervous   c. lymphoid
    b. cartilage   d. skin

40. Which of the following is formed as a consequence of the indirect effect of radiation?

    a. free radicals   c. DNA
    b. water   d. proteins

41. Which of the following graphs is identified as semilog?

    a. A   c. C
    b. B   d. D

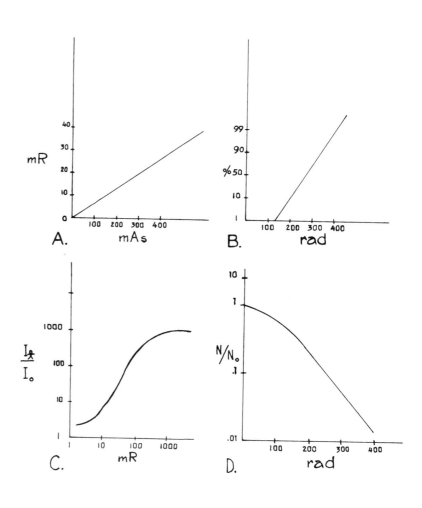

42. Which of the following is considered a late radiation response?

   a. cataracts
   b. moist desquamation
   c. lymphocytic depression
   d. epilation

43. Which region of this multitarget, single-hit cell survival curve represents the target number?

   a. A   c. C
   b. B   d. D

44. Approximately how many American females develop breast cancer?

   a. 1%   c. 10%
   b. 5%   d. 20%

45. Which of the following human responses to radiation exposure is deterministic?

   a. breast cancer
   b. life-span shortening
   c. skin erythema
   d. skin cancer

46. Which of the following radiation-induced effects is stochastic?

   a. cataracts   c. skin erythema
   b. breast cancer   d. epilation

47. Radiation-induced cataracts

   a. appear on the anterior pole of the lens.
   b. appear on the posterior pole of the lens.
   c. follow a linear, nonthreshold dose-response relationship.
   d. follow a nonlinear, nonthreshold relationship.

48. X-ray mammography requires approximately 100 mrad per view. What is the approximate risk of developing breast cancer from such an examination?

   a. 1 in 100   c. 1 in 10,000
   b. 1 in 1,000   d. 1 in 100,000

49. Approximately what minimal dose is required to produce an erythema on the hands of an angiointerventional radiologist?

   a. 50 rad   c. 300 rad
   b. 100 rad   d. 600 rad

50. Which of the following populations have experienced an excessive incidence of leukemia?

   a. radium watch dial painters
   b. uranium miners
   c. TB fluoroscopy patients
   d. atomic bomb survivors

51. Which of the following is the best measure of cellular radiosensitivity?

   a. $LD_{50/30}$ c. D_Q
   b. D_0 d. target number n

52. Atrophy is a term that relates to tissue
    a. enlargement.
    b. shrinkage.
    c. radiosensitivity.
    d. radiation resistance.

53. Which of the following chromosome aberrations is of the multihit type?
    a. ring chromosome
    b. isochromatid deletion
    c. chromatid deletion
    d. chromatid break

54. A deterministic effect refers to
    a. early effects of human responses to radiation exposure.
    b. late effects of human responses to radiation exposure.
    c. acute high-dose radiation exposure.
    d. protracted low-dose radiation exposure.

55. The $LD_{50/30}$ for humans is approximately
    a. 100 rad.
    b. 350 rad.
    c. 500 rad.
    d. 800 rad.

56. A relative risk of 2:1 means
    a. two radiation-induced cases of disease.
    b. twice as many cases of disease as expected.
    c. a 200% increase in incidence.
    d. two cases per 100,000/year/rad.

57. Which of the following blood cell types is most sensitive to radiation exposure?
    a. red blood cells
    b. platelets
    c. neutrophils
    d. lymphocytes

58. Which of the following radiation-induced effects is stochastic?
    a. death
    b. life shortening
    c. moist desquamation
    d. leukemia

59. Approximately what dose of occupational x-ray exposure is necessary to produce cataracts?
    a. 10 rad
    b. 100 rad
    c. 1,000 rad
    d. 10,000 rad

60. Which of the following populations has experienced an excessive incidence of bone cancer?
    a. radium watch dial painters
    b. uranium miners
    c. TB fluoroscopy patients
    d. atomic bomb survivors

61. ALARA stands for
    a. a lovely afternoon reading action
    b. at last a real anatomy
    c. as long as rads attend
    d. as low as reasonably achievable

62. In general, when evaluating cellular radiosensitivity,
    a. cells with a high D_0 are more sensitive.
    b. cells with higher target numbers are more sensitive.
    c. cells with a higher D_Q are more sensitive.
    d. oxygenated cells are more sensitive.

63. Which of the following is the most radiosensitive tissue?
    a. nervous   c. lymphoid
    b. cartilage   d. skin

64. Which type of chromosomal aberration requires karyotypic analysis for detection?
    a. ring chromosome
    b. reciprocal translocation
    c. isochromatid break
    d. dicentric chromosome

65. When radiation effects are termed deterministic,
    a. they occur soon after exposure.
    b. they occur many years after exposure.
    c. the severity of the response is dose-related.
    d. the incidence of the response is dose-related.

66. The minimum dose of x rays that will produce a skin erythema when delivered acutely is approximately
    a. 50 rad.   c. 200 rad.
    b. 100 rad.   d. 400 rad.

67. Which of the following describes a stochastic effect of radiation?
    a. a low-threshold dose
    b. no threshold dose
    c. a whole-body effect
    d. an organ or tissue effect

68. Which of the following represents the single-target, single-hit radiation dose-response relationship for cell lethality?
    a. A   c. C
    b. B   d. D

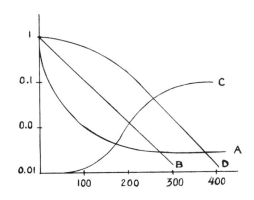

69. The sequence of events following radiation exposure proceed from
    a. bond disruption to cellular transformation biochemical alteration to whole-body effects.
    b. bond disruption to biochemical alteration to whole-body effects to cellular transformation.
    c. ionization to bond disruption to biochemical alteration to cell transformation.
    d. ionization to biochemical alteration to bond disruption to cell transformation.

70. Which of the following molecules **is least** abundant in the human body?
    a. water   c. proteins
    b. carbohydrates   d. nucleic acids

71. If electron excitation were the only radiation interaction with tissue, the principal result would be
    a. ionization.   c. light.
    b. heat.   d. bond disruption.

72. When water is irradiated, a principal molecular product is
    a. ionization.   c. nucleic acids.
    b. excitation.   d. free radicals.

73. Free radicals are
    a. long-lived molecules.
    b. energetic molecules.
    c. harmless molecules.
    d. biochemical bonds.

74. Which of the following **is not** a measure of human cell radiosensitivity?
    a. D_0 c. D_{37}
    b. D_Q d. $LD_{50/30}$

75. If ionizing radiation interacted with DNA, it would be called
    a. a direct effect.   c. transformation.
    b. an indirect effect. d. bond disruption.

76. In this example of a multitarget, single-hit cell survival curve, which region represents D_Q?
    a. A   c. C
    b. B   d. D

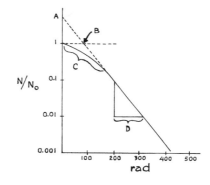

77. As time increases following radiation exposure,

    a. the single-hit/multihit ratio of chromosomal aberrations increases.
    b. the single-hit/multihit ratio of chromosomal aberrations decreases.
    c. the number of chromosomal aberrations increases.
    d. the chromosomal aberration rate decreases to zero.

78. What minimum acute radiation dose results in sterility?

    a. 50 rad   c. 5,000 rad
    b. 500 rad   d. 50,000 rad

79. Which of the following is a deterministic effect?

    a. breast cancer   c. genetic mutations
    b. leukemia   d. cataracts

80. Which of the following represents the multitarget, single-hit radiation dose-response relationship for cell lethality?

    a. A   c. C
    b. B   d. D

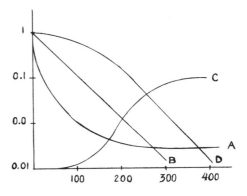

81. Which radiation dose-response relationship describes the irradiation of human cells in vivo?

    a. single-target, single-hit
    b. single-target, multihit
    c. multitarget, single-hit
    d. multitarget, multihit

82. When only the nucleus is irradiated, the dose required to kill a cell is approximately

    a. 10 rad.   c. 1,000 rad.
    b. 100 rad.   d. 10,000 rad.

83. When radiation interacts with human cells, the interaction is

    a. uniform.   c. linear.
    b. random.   d. quadratic.

84. Which of the following is a stochastic effect?

    1. lung cancer   a. Only 1, 2, and 3 are correct.
    2. sterility   b. Only 1 and 3 are correct.
    3. genetic mutations   c. Only 2 and 4 are correct.
    4. cataracts   d. All are correct.

85. If radiation interacted uniformly for the single-target, single-hit radiation dose-response relationship, a dose equal to D_{37} would kill what fraction of cells?

    a. 0%
    b. 37%
    c. 63%
    d. 100%

86. Our best estimate for radiation-induced life-span shortening is

    a. 0.1 d/rad.
    b. 1.0 d/rad.
    c. 10 d/rad.
    d. 100 d/rad.

87. One human response to radiation that can be distinguished from that occurring naturally is

    a. cataracts.
    b. leukemia.
    c. breast cancer.
    d. moist desquamation.

88. The risk that radiation will induce cancer or leukemia following a dose of 1 rad is approximately

    a. 1 in 100.
    b. 1 in 1,000.
    c. 1 in 10,000.
    d. 1 in 100,000.

89. Which of the following populations have experienced an excessive incidence of lung cancer?

    a. radium watch dial painters
    b. uranium miners
    c. TB fluoroscopy patients
    d. atomic bomb survivors

90. During which period of pregnancy will high irradiation of the embryo or fetus most likely result in a congenital abnormality?

    a. the first 2 weeks
    b. weeks 3 to 10
    c. the second trimester
    d. the third trimester

91. In general, when evaluating cellular radiosensitivity,

    a. cells with a high D_0 are more sensitive.
    b. cells with low target numbers are more sensitive.
    c. cells with a higher D_Q are more sensitive.
    d. anoxic cells are more sensitive.

92. Which of the following molecules are most abundant in the human body?

    a. water
    b. carbohydrates
    c. proteins
    d. nucleic acids

93. Which of the following is considered a single-hit chromosomal aberration?

    a. ring chromosome
    b. isochromatid
    c. dicentric
    d. reciprocal translocation

94. The term **karyotype** refers to the mapping of each chromosome in a cell according to its

    a. sex.
    b. size.
    c. number.
    d. color.

95. Which of the following human responses to radiation exposure is an early effect?
    a. epilation
    b. leukemia
    c. bone cancer
    d. cataracts

96. The minimum radiation dose required to produce tissue or organ atrophy is approximately
    a. 100 rad.
    b. 250 rad.
    c. 500 rad.
    d. 1,000 rad.

97. When evaluating relative cell radiosensitivity, cells irradiated
    1. with high-LET radiation are more sensitive than those treated with low-LET radiation.
    2. with a fractionated dose are more sensitive than those treated with an acute dose.
    3. in the presence of oxygen are more sensitive than those treated in the presence of nitrogen.
    4. at a reduced dose rate are more sensitive than if irradiated acutely.
    a. Only 1, 2, and 3 are correct.
    b. Only 1 and 3 are correct.
    c. Only 2 and 4 are correct.
    d. Only 4 is correct.

98. Which of the following populations have experienced an excessive incidence of breast cancer?
    1. radium watch dial painters
    2. atomic bomb survivors
    3. uranium miners
    4. TB fluoroscopy patients
    a. Only 1, 2, and 3 are correct.
    b. Only 1 and 3 are correct.
    c. Only 2 and 4 are correct.
    d. Only 4 is correct.

99. A patient undergoes several CT examinations of the head, receiving a lens dose of 25 rad. What is the probability of cataract formation because of this dose?
    a. 0%
    b. 0.1%
    c. 1.0%
    d. 10%

100. When evaluating relative cell radiosensitivity, cells irradiated
    1. with high-LET radiation are more sensitive than those treated with low-LET radiation.
    2. in the presence of those treated in the presence of nitrogen.
    3. with a fractionated dose are less sensitive than those treated with an acute dose.
    4. at a reduced dose rate are less sensitive than if irradiated with an acute dose.
    a. Only 1, 2, and 3 are correct.
    b. Only 1 and 3 are correct.
    c. Only 2 and 4 are correct.
    d. All are correct.

101. Which of the following is a distinctive and characteristic radiation effect?

    a. Thyroid cancer induced by ^{131}I is of a different type than that caused by x rays.

    b. Breast cancer in radium watch dial painters is different from that seen in atomic bomb survivors.

    c. Cataracts induced by radiation form on the posterior pole of the lens.

    d. Genetic effects caused by radiation are easily distinguished from those that occur naturally.

102. Which of the following tissues is most sensitive to x-ray exposure?

    a. skin   c. thyroid

    b. gonads   d. lens

103. Nausea is principally associated with

    a. prodromal syndrome.

    b. the latent period.

    c. hematological syndrome.

    d. gastrointestinal syndrome.

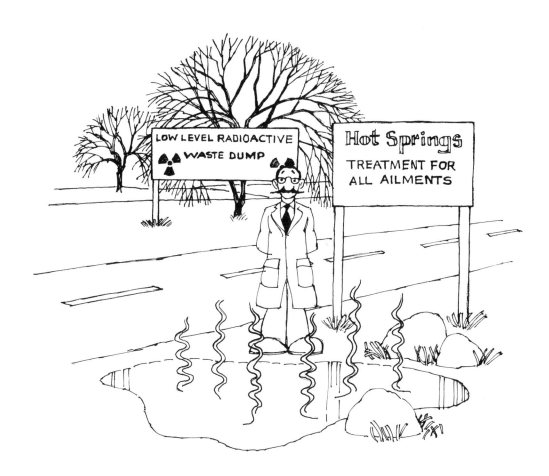

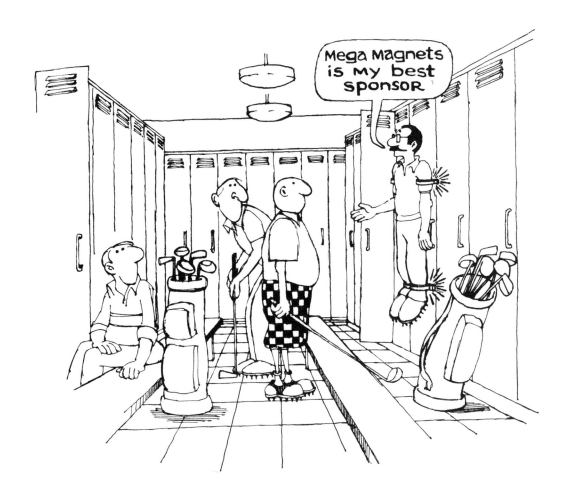

Patient Radiation Control

- The cardinal principles of radiation protection—reduce time, increase distance, use shielding—apply especially to radiology patients.

- The measure of patient dose is that to the skin—entrance skin exposure (ESE).

- ESE is easy to measure using radiation dosimeters.

- ESE is relatively easy to estimate by computation.

- ESE increases proportionately with increasing mAs.

- ESE increases quadratically with increasing kVp, that is, proportionately with increasing kVp^2.

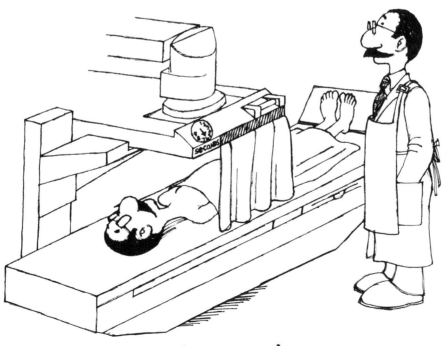

⇩ Time, ⇧ Distance, ⇧ shielding

Approximate Entrance Skin Exposure

PA chest   —   10 mrad
extremity   —   10 mrad
lateral skull   —   70 mrad
shoulder   —   80 mrad
cervical spine —   110 mrad
thoracic spine —   180 mrad
abdomen   —   220 mrad

Patient dose is reduced by

using high kVp technique
maintaining processor QC
x-ray beam filtration
using long SID
avoiding retakes
x-ray beam collimation
using gonad shields

Always use gonad shields
for radiographs of:

Pelvis

Hip (except oblique
        views)

Upper Femur

- In general, a high-kVp examination results in a lower ESE because much less mAs is required.

- Rule of thumb: ESE = 5 mR/mAs.

- ESE increases quadratically (Inverse Square Law) as source-to-skin distance (SSD) is reduced.

- If mR/mAs is known at a given kVp from a medical physicist's report, ESE can be computed for any technique.

- Patient dose can be reduced by maintaining proper darkroom, processing, and quality control procedures.

- Patient dose during radiography can be reduced by using a high-kVp technique.

- Patient dose during radiography can be reduced by adding filtration to the primary beam.

- Patient dose during radiography can be reduced by using a long source-to-image-receptor distance (SID).

- Patient dose during radiography can be reduced by using faster image receptors.

- Patient dose during radiography can be reduced most effectively by avoiding retakes.

- Collimation during radiography and fluoroscopy is an application of shielding for patient radiation protection.

- An added benefit of collimation is the reduction of scatter radiation, resulting in improved image contrast.

- Positive beam limitation (PBL) is a method of automatic collimation.

- Patient dose during radiography can be reduced by using gonadal shields.

- Gonadal shields should be used on all patients of childbearing age when the use of such shields will not interfere with obtaining the required diagnostic information and the useful beam is within 5 cm of the gonads.

- During fluoroscopy, patient dose is principally determined by the on time of the x-ray beam.

- During fluoroscopy, ESE is approximately 4,000 mR/min.

- During fluoroscopy, ESE increases proportionately with the number of spot films.

- During fluoroscopy, ESE is approximately 200 mR per view for cassette-loaded spot films.

- During fluoroscopy, ESE is approximately 100 mR per view for photospots.

- During fluoroscopy, ESE is approximately 200 mR per frame for digital fluoroscopy.

- ESE is approximately 1,000 mR/s for cineradiography at 15 frames/s.

- ESE increases proportionately with increasing frame rate during cineradiography.

- Organ dose can be estimated and is a good predictor of biological response.

- Mean marrow dose (MMD) is the average dose to the active bone marrow. MMD is a predictor of radiation-induced leukemia.

- MMD from medical x-ray imaging is approximately 100 mrad/y.

- The average effective dose (E) from medical x-ray imaging is approximately 50 mrem/y.

- Genetically significant dose (GSD) is the average dose to the gonads of patients of reproductive age.

- GSD is a predictor of radiation-induced genetic mutations.

- GSD from medical x-ray imaging is estimated to be 20 mrad/y.

- Mean glandular dose (D_G) is the dose to the glandular tissue of the breast.

- D_G is used as a predictor of radiation-induced breast cancer.

- D_G is approximately 100 mrad per view for nongrid mammography.

- D_G is approximately 200 mrad per view for grid mammography.

- D_G is approximately 200 mrad per view for magnification mammography without a grid.

- Patient dose during computed tomography (CT) is essentially uniform from skin to midline.

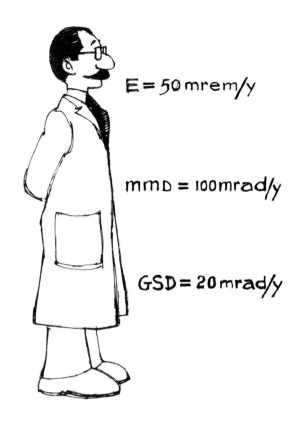

$$E = 50\,mrem/y$$

$$mmD = 100\,mrad/y$$

$$GSD = 20\,mrad/y$$

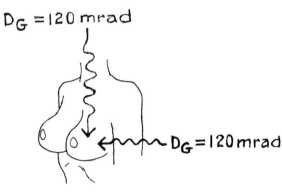

$$D_G = 120\,mrad$$

$$D_G = 120\,mrad$$

$$Total\ D_G = 240\,mrad$$

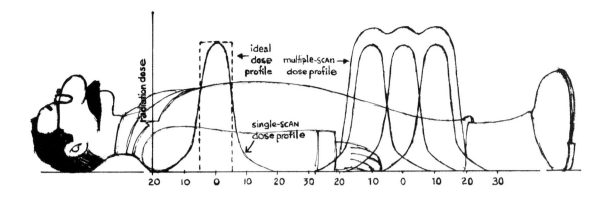

- During CT, sequential images require irradiation of different tissue and dose is therefore unrelated to the number of scans.

- Patient dose during CT is approximately 5,000 mrad per scan.

- Patient dose for a complete CT examination is approximately 10% higher than that for a single-slice examination.

- Patient dose during spiral CT is lower for a higher pitch.

- Patient dose during radiography is proportional to the number of views.

- Patient dose during fluoroscopy is proportional to the fluoroscopy time.

- A routine chest x-ray should not be performed as part of the admission of hospital patients.

- A chest x-ray examination should not be performed on asymptomatic patients during routine medical examinations.

- A chest x-ray should not be performed as a screening test for tuberculosis.

- Fluoroscopy should not be performed on asymptomatic patients as a part of routine medical examinations.

- During fluoroscopy, the technologist must note the examination time and technique for each patient examination.

- During radiography, the use of fast intensifying screens reduces patient dose.

- During radiography, patient dose is inversely proportional to radiographic intensifying screen speed.

- Pregnant patients can be examined radiographically or fluoroscopically if the examination is necessary for proper patient management.

- The ALARA philosophy (**as low as reasonably achievable**) should be instituted for patients as well as personnel.

Chapter 6 Practice Questions

1. The cardinal principles of radiation control include
   1. distance.
   2. shielding.
   3. time.
   4. occupation.
   a. Only 1, 2 and 3 are correct.
   b. Only 1 and 3 are correct.
   c. Only 2 and 4 are correct.
   d. All are correct.

2. As a general rule of thumb, if one wishes to estimate entrance skin exposure, one should assume a radiation intensity at the skin of approximately
   a. 2 mR/mAs.   c. 20 mR/mAs.
   b. 5 mR/mAs.   d. 50 mR/mAs.

3. A 30-slice CT examination is obtained with and without contrast media. The approximate patient dose is
   a. 1,000 mrad.   c. 10,000 mrad.
   b. 5,000 mrad.   d. 20,000 mrad.

4. A Townes view is obtained at 68 kVp/80 mAs. The approximate entrance skin exposure is
   a. 20 mR.   c. 200 mR.
   b. 40 mR.   d. 400 mR.

5. Which of the following conditions requires the use of gonadal shields?
   1. if the patient is of childbearing age
   2. if the image receptor speed is less than 100
   3. if the gonads are within 5 cm of the useful beam
   4. if the shield is large enough to cover the abdomen and pelvis
   a. Only 1, 2 and 3 are correct.
   b. Only 1 and 3 are correct.
   c. Only 2 and 4 are correct.
   d. All are correct.

6. During fluoroscopic examination, patient dose is
   1. proportional to x-ray beam time.
   2. proportional to examination time.
   3. proportional to the number of spot films.
   4. proportional to image intensifier size.
   a. Only 1, 2, and 3 are correct.
   b. Only 1 and 3 are correct.
   c. Only 2 and 4 are correct.
   d. All are correct.

7. Patient dose for a single CT scan is 5,000 mrad. What is the total dose for a patient who has a 20-section CT examination?
   a. 5,000 mrad   c. 10,000 mrad
   b. 5,500 mrad   d. 100,000 mrad

8. During a fluoroscopic examination, 16 photospot views are obtained. What is the approximate patient entrance skin exposure due to these spot views?
   a. 200 mR   c. 1,200 mR
   b. 800 mR   d. 1,600 mR

9. The individual mean marrow dose due to diagnostic x-ray imaging is approximately
   a. 100 mrad/y.   c. 400 mrad/y.
   b. 200 mrad/y.   d. 800 mrad/y.

10. During spiral CT, if one increases the pitch of the examination, patient dose will
    a. be reduced.
    b. remain approximately the same.
    c. be increased.
    d. be very much increased.

11. As an approximation, patient dose during computed tomography is
    a. 1,000 mrad.   c. 10,000 mrad.
    b. 5,000 mrad.   d. 20,000 mrad.

12. Which of the following techniques will result in reduced patient dose?
    1. notation of time and technique during fluoroscopy
    2. use of fast radiographic intensifying screens
    3. reducing image intensifier size
    4. reducing fluoroscopic x-ray beam time

a. Only 1, 2 and 3 are correct.
b. Only 1 and 3 are correct.
c. Only 2 and 4 are correct.
d. All are correct.

13. Of the following measures of patient dose, which is the easiest to measure directly?

a. organ dose
b. entrance skin exposure
c. integral dose
d. genetic dose

14. Which of the following is appropriate for an ALARA program?

a. issuing a temporary radiation monitor to each patient
b. performing a periodic review of diagnostic accuracy
c. analyzing rejected films for cause of rejection
d. using the fastest image receptors regardless of image quality

15. As the SID is increased while radiographic technique **remains fixed**, entrance skin exposure

a. decreases according to the inverse square law.
b. decreases proportionately.
c. increases proportionately.
d. increases according to the inverse square law.

16. A KUB (kidneys, ureters, bladder) examination is performed at 76 kVp/30 mAs. What is the approximate entrance skin exposure?

a. 30 mR   c. 150 mR
b. 75 mR   d. 300 mR

17. For which of the following situations is a chest x-ray examination contraindicated?

1. hospital admission of all patients
2. as part of an annual physical
3. annually for food handlers
4. in screening for tuberculosis

a. Only 1, 2 and 3 are correct.
b. Only 1 and 3 are correct.
c. Only 2 and 4 are correct.
d. All are correct.

18. Which of the following conditions requires the use of gonadal shields?

1. if the patient is a male of any age
2. if the gonads are in the useful beam
3. if the image receptor is too slow
4. if use of such shields does not interfere with obtaining the required diagnostic information

a. Only 1, 2 and 3 are correct.
b. Only 1 and 3 are correct.
c. Only 2 and 4 are correct.
d. All are correct.

19. During fluoroscopic examination, patient dose is proportional to

    1. examination time.
    2. image intensifier size.
    3. spot film size.
    4. mA.

    a. Only 1, 2 and 3 are correct.
    b. Only 1 and 3 are correct.
    c. Only 2 and 4 are correct.
    d. Only 4 is correct.

20. During a fluoroscopic examination, 25 digital views are obtained. What is the approximate patient entrance skin exposure due to these views?

    a. 1,000 mR   c. 10,000 mR
    b. 5,000 mR   d. 50,000 mR

21. If a 26-year-old patient whose last menstrual period was 3 weeks ago is referred for barium enema examination, one should

    a. perform the examination according to ALARA.
    b. perform the examination according to the 10-day rule.
    c. wait until the next menstrual period.
    d. wait until pregnancy is ruled out.

22. The annual genetically significant dose per person is estimated to be approximately

    a. 5 mrad.   c. 20 mrad.
    b. 10 mrad.   d. 50 mrad.

23. A head CT examination is performed at 120 kVp/400 mA and 20 slices are obtained. The approximate patient dose is

    a. 2,000 mrad.   c. 20,000 mrad.
    b. 5,000 mrad.   d. 50,000 mrad.

24. Which of the following techniques will result in reduced patient dose?

    1. collimation of x-ray beam
    2. use of single-emulsion film
    3. restricting the number of fluoroscopic spot films
    4. reducing fluoroscopic examination time

    a. Only 1, 2, and 3 are correct.
    b. Only 1 and 3 are correct.
    c. Only 2 and 4 are correct.
    d. All are correct.

25. Patient dose is

    a. inversely related to mAs.
    b. independent of mAs.
    c. proportional to mAs.
    d. proportional to mAs^2.

26. As the SID is increased with a **compensating change in radiographic technique** to maintain acceptable image quality, the entrance skin exposure

    a. decreases according to the inverse square law.
    b. decreases.
    c. increases.
    d. increases according to the inverse square law.

27. A posterior-anterior (PA) chest examination is conducted at 110 kVp/3 mAs. What is the approximate entrance skin exposure?

    a. 10 mR   c. 20 mR
    b. 15 mR   d. 30 mR

28. Patient dose during a fluoroscopic exam is principally determined by

    a. examination time.
    b. x-ray beam time.
    c. kVp of operation.
    d. size of the image intensifier tube.

29. During fluoroscopy, patient entrance skin exposure from cassette-loaded spot films is approximately

    a. 100 mR per view.
    b. 200 mR per view.
    c. 500 mR per view.
    d. 1,000 mR per view.

30. Which of the following techniques will result in reduced patient dose?

    1. notation of time and technique during fluoroscopy
    2. use of fast radiographic intensifying screens
    3. removal of added filtration
    4. reducing on time of the fluoroscopic x-ray beam

    a. Only 1, 2, and 3 are correct.
    b. Only 1 and 3 are correct.
    c. Only 2 and 4 are correct.
    d. All are correct.

31. During a cardiac catheterization, 15 s of cineradiography at 30 frames/s is performed. What is the approximate patient entrance skin exposure due to this cineradiography?

    a. 15,000 mR   c. 150,000 mR
    b. 30,000 mR   d. 300,000 mR

32. During mammography using a grid, the mean glandular dose per view is approximately

    a. 50 mrad.   c. 200 mrad.
    b. 100 mrad.   d. 400 mrad.

33. An abdominal CT exam is conducted at 125 kVp/300 mA and 30 slices are obtained. The approximate patient dose is

    a. 3,000 mrad.   c. 30,000 mrad.
    b. 5,000 mrad.   d. 50,000 mrad.

34. Which of the following techniques will result in reduced patient dose?
    1. using the largest image intensifier mode
    2. using fast image receptors
    3. restricting cineradiographic time
    4. reducing kVp of examination
    a. Only 1, 2, and 3 are correct.
    b. Only 1 and 3 are correct.
    c. Only 2 and 4 are correct.
    d. All are correct.

35. Patient dose is
    a. inversely proportional to kVp.
    b. independent of kVp.
    c. proportional to kVp.
    d. proportional to kVp^2.

36. A KUB examination is performed at 74 kVp/40 mAs. What is the approximate entrance skin exposure?
    a. 5 mR   c. 100 mR
    b. 40 mR   d. 200 mR

37. A PA spine exam is obtained at 72 kVp/60 mAs. What is the approximate entrance skin exposure?
    a. 150 mR   c. 600 mR
    b. 300 mR   d. 1,200 mR

38. The entrance skin exposure during fluoroscopy is approximately
    a. 1,000 mR/min.   c. 4,000 mR/min.
    b. 2,000 mR/min.   d. 8,000 mR/min.

39. During fluoroscopy, patient entrance skin exposure from photospot images is approximately
    a. 100 mR per view.   c. 500 mR per view.
    b. 200 mR per view.   d. 1,000 mR per view.

40. Which of the following is used as a predictor of radiation-induced leukemia?
    a. mean marrow dose
    b. genetically significant dose
    c. mean glandular dose
    d. entrance skin exposure

41. During mammography without a grid, the mean glandular dose per view is approximately
    a. 50 mrad.   c. 200 mrad.
    b. 100 mrad.   d. 400 mrad.

42. A 10-slice CT scan examination is obtained and repeated with contrast media. The approximate patient dose is
    a. 2,000 mrad.   c. 10,000 mrad.
    b. 5,000 mrad.   d. 20,000 mrad.

43. Which of the following techniques will result in reduced patient dose?

    1. using high-kVp radiographic technique
    2. using nonscreen film
    3. restricting the number of fluoroscopic spot films
    4. resetting the 5-min fluoroscopy timer

    a. Only 1, 2, and 3 are correct.
    b. Only 1 and 3 are correct.
    c. Only 2 and 4 are correct.
    d. All are correct.

44. When comparing several acceptable radiographs, the technique that usually results in lower patient dose is that based on

    a. reduced SID.
    b. reduced beam filtration.
    c. increased mAs.
    d. increased kVp.

45. A PA chest examination is conducted at 110 kVp/3 mAs. What is the approximate entrance skin exposure?

    a. 1 mR   c. 10 mR
    b. 5 mR   d. 50 mR

46. A Townes view is obtained at 66 kVp/65 mAs. The approximate entrance skin exposure is

    a. 40 mR.   c. 160 mR.
    b. 80 mR.   d. 320 mR.

47. A barium enema examination is conducted at approximately 90 kVp and 2.5 mA and requires 1.5 min x-ray beam time. What is the approximate entrance skin exposure?

    a. 6,000 mR   c. 20,000 mR
    b. 12,000 mR   d. 40,000 mR

48. During fluoroscopy, patient entrance skin exposure from digital images is approximately

    a. 100 mR per frame.   c. 500 mR per frame.
    b. 200 mR per frame.   d. 1,000 mR per frame.

49. Which of the following is used as a predictor of radiation-induced genetic mutations?

    a. mean marrow dose.
    b. genetically significant dose.
    c. mean glandular dose.
    d. entrance skin exposure.

50. During magnification mammography, the mean glandular dose per view is approximately

    a. 50 mrad.   c. 200 mrad.
    b. 100 mrad.   d. 400 mrad.

51. Which of the following techniques will result in reduced patient dose?
    1. collimation to body part
    2. switching to an unmagnified fluoroscopy view
    3. replacing cassette spot films with photospot films
    4. reducing on time of fluoroscopic x-ray beam

    a. Only 1, 2, and 3 are correct.
    b. Only 1 and 3 are correct.
    c. Only 2 and 4 are correct.
    d. All are correct.

52. During spiral CT, when one increases the pitch of the examination, patient dose is

    a. reduced.
    b. remains approximately the same.
    c. increased.
    d. very much increased.

53. When comparing acceptable radiographs, which of the following techniques usually results in reduced patient dose?
    1. increased SID
    2. increased filtration
    3. increased kVp
    4. increased mAs

    a. Only 1, 2, and 3 are correct.
    b. Only 1 and 3 are correct.
    c. Only 2 and 4 are correct.
    d. All are correct.

54. A lateral spine exam is obtained at 78 kVp/120 mAs. What is the approximate entrance skin exposure?

    a. 5 mR   c. 500 mR
    b. 50 mR   d. 5,000 mR

55. The greatest reduction in patient dose is obtained by

    a. using high-kVp technique.
    b. using long-SID technique.
    c. shielding the patient appropriately.
    d. avoiding retakes.

56. Gonadal shields are required for some patients in order to reduce the

    a. probability of transient infertility.
    b. probability of sterility.
    c. probability of genetic mutations.
    d. population genetically significant dose.

57. The estimated value of the genetically significant dose is

    a. 20 mrad/y.   c. 100 mrad/y.
    b. 50 mrad/y.   d. 200 mrad/y.

58. Which of the following is an application of ALARA for patients?

    a. issuing each patient a film badge
    b. employing high-mAs technique
    c. applying gonad shields when appropriate
    d. delaying radiographic examination of pregnant patients

59. Which of the following conditions requires the use of gonadal shields?

    1. if the patient is of childbearing age
    2. if the gonads are in the useful beam
    3. if the gonads are within 5 cm of the useful beam
    4. if the shields are made of lead or lead equivalent

    a. Only 1, 2, and 3 are correct.
    b. Only 1 and 3 are correct.
    c. Only 2 and 4 are correct.
    d. All are correct.

60. A coronary artery angioplasty requires 22 min of x-ray beam time. What is the approximate entrance skin exposure?

    a. 22,000 mR
    b. 88,000 mR
    c. 144,000 mR
    d. 166,000 mR

61. During a fluoroscopic examination, eight cassette-loaded spot views are obtained. What is the approximate patient entrance skin exposure due to these spot views?

    a. 200 mR
    b. 800 mR
    c. 1,200 mR
    d. 1,600 mR

62. Which of the following is used as a predictor of radiation-induced erythema?

    a. mean marrow dose
    b. genetically significant dose
    c. mean glandular dose
    d. entrance skin exposure

63. When compared with that for a single-section examination, patient dose during a 15-section computed tomography examination is

    a. equal.
    b. slightly higher.
    c. approximately twice as high.
    d. approximately 15 times as high.

64. A chest x-ray examination is contraindicated for which of the following situations?

    1. hospital admission of a patient with cardiac distress
    2. part of an annual physical
    3. upper respiratory infection in the elderly
    4. screening for tuberculosis

    a. Only 1, 2, and 3 are correct.
    b. Only 1 and 3 are correct.
    c. Only 2 and 4 are correct.
    d. All are correct.

65. A cerebral angiogram requires approximately 12 min of x-ray beam time. What is the approximate entrance skin exposure?
    a. 50,000 mR
    b. 100,000 mR
    c. 200,000 mR
    d. 400,000 mR

66. Which of the following techniques will result in reduced patient dose?
    1. adding x-ray beam filtration
    2. collimating to body part
    3. using high-kVp technique
    4. remaining behind the control booth barrier
    a. Only 1, 2 and 3 are correct.
    b. Only 1 and 3 are correct.
    c. Only 2 and 4 are correct.
    d. All are correct.

67. During fluoroscopy, patient entrance skin exposure during cineradiography at 15 frames/s is approximately
    a. 100 mR/s.
    b. 200 mR/s.
    c. 500 mR/s.
    d. 1,000 mR/s.

68. Which of the following is used as a predictor of radiation-induced breast cancer?
    a. mean marrow dose
    b. genetically significant dose
    c. mean glandular dose
    d. entrance skin exposure

69. During computed tomography, the midline dose is
    a. very much less than the skin dose.
    b. approximately equal to the skin dose.
    c. very much more than the skin dose.
    d. varies greatly with the skin dose according to the type of examination.

70. Entrance skin exposure (ESE) during a PA chest radiograph is approximately
    a. 10 mR.
    b. 50 mR.
    c. 100 mR.
    d. 500 mR.

71. What radiation device is unique to C-arm fluoroscopy?
    a. buck slot cover
    b. spacer
    c. dead man switch
    d. cumulative timer

72. The 10-day rule
    a. applies to the 10 days before menstruation.
    b. applies to the period of menstruation.
    c. should be vigorously observed.
    d. has been abandoned.

73. During fluoroscopy, the tabletop exposure rate must not exceed
    a. 1 R/min.
    b. 10 R/min.
    c. 10 R/h.
    d. 100 R/h.

Occupational Radiation Control

- Occupational radiation exposure in x-ray imaging is exceedingly low.

- We receive most of our occupational radiation exposure during fluoroscopy.

- During radiography the technician should remain behind the control booth.

- During radiography the technician should fix the exposure control to the operating console so that he cannot stand outside the control booth.

- During radiography the technician should never direct the useful beam at the control booth.

- Rule of thumb: Occupational radiation exposure during table-side fluoroscopy is approximately 1 mrem/min.

- During fluoroscopy, protective gloves and an apron must be worn.

- During fluoroscopy, protective apparel reduces radiation exposure to the protected parts of the body to near zero.

- Approximately half of all radiologic technologists receive no measurable occupational exposure each year.

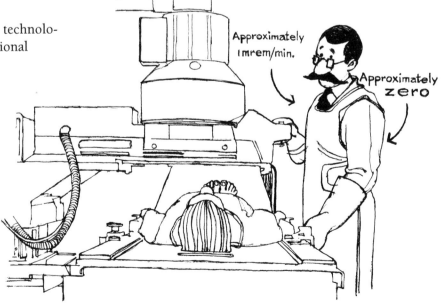

Approximately 1mrem/min.

Approximately zero

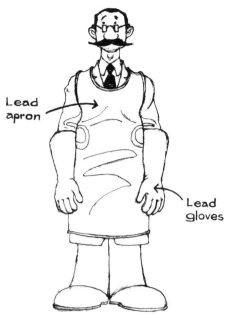

Lead apron

Lead gloves

Required Protective Apparel

- The average dose equivalent to a radiologic technologist in the United States is approximately 50 mrem/y.

- Pregnant physicians and radiologic technologists present special problems.

- Practicing normal radiation control procedures during pregnancy ensures a safe working environment.

- Pregnancy is no reason to avoid fluoroscopy.

- Protective apparel of at least 0.5 mm lead equivalent should be worn during fluoroscopy.

- Obey the cardinal principles of radiation protection at all times: Reduce exposure time, increase distance from source, and use shielding where appropriate.

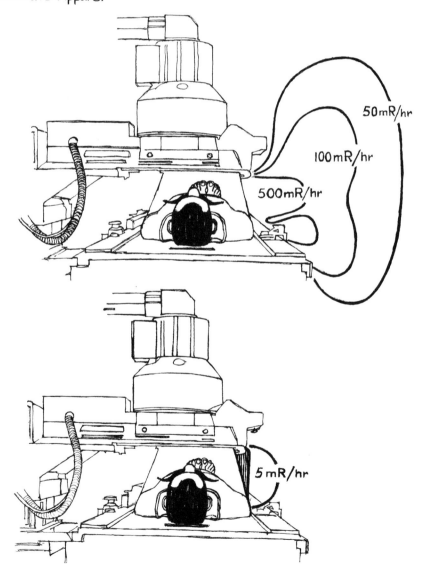

50 mR/hr

100 mR/hr

500 mR/hr

5 mR/hr

- During fluoroscopy, when possible, take one or more steps back from the table. Radiation exposure falls off sharply from table side.

- During fluoroscopy, the patient becomes the principal source of radiation exposure due to scatter radiation.

- During C-arm fluoroscopy position the x-ray tube below the patient.

- During fluoroscopy, position your occupational radiation monitor, film badge, or other device at the collar, outside the protective apron.

- During pregnancy, a second occupational radiation monitor should be positioned at waist level under the protective apron.

- The second monitor worn during pregnancy should be color-coded and identified as a baby badge.

- Take special care not to switch a body badge with a baby badge.

- An ALARA (as low as reasonably achievable) program should be a part of any personnel radiation control program.

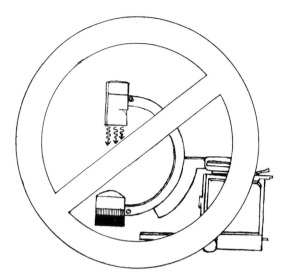

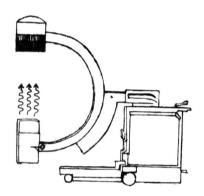

Chapter 7 Practice Questions

1. In diagnostic imaging, most occupational radiation exposure is received during
   a. radiography.
   b. fluoroscopy.
   c. computed tomography.
   d. mammography.

2. During fluoroscopy, the protective lead apron reduces exposure to the trunk of the body to approximately what percentage shown on a collar-positioned occupational radiation monitor?
   a. 0
   b. 5
   c. 25
   d. 50

3. In order to reduce occupational radiation exposure, the following practices are helpful
   1. reducing fluoroscopic x-ray beam time
   2. wearing protective apparel during fluoroscopy
   3. remaining behind the control booth barrier during radiography
   4. maintaining as much distance as possible from an angiointerventional patient

   a. Only 1, 2 and 3 are correct.
   b. Only 1 and 3 are correct.
   c. Only 2 and 4 are correct.
   d. All are correct.

4. During fluoroscopy, the principal source of occupational radiation exposure is
   a. the patient.
   b. leakage radiation from the x-ray tube under the table.
   c. scatter radiation from the walls.
   d. transmitted radiation through the image intensifier tube.

5. Which of the following is an appropriate radiation protection measure to be implemented **only during pregnancy?**
   1. reassignment to nonradiation work
   2. wearing a thicker protective apron
   3. exchanging radiation monitors weekly
   4. instituting fetal monitoring with a second radiation monitor
   a. Only 1, 2, and 3 are correct.
   b. Only 1 and 3 are correct.
   c. Only 2 and 4 are correct.
   d. Only 4 is correct.

6. Which of the following is appropriate to an ALARA program for radiologists and radiographers?
   a. performing daily monitoring of a film processor
   b. using high-kVp radiographic technique
   c. formally investigating any abnormally high film badge reading
   d. providing two film badges to each employee

7. Protective apparel should be worn
   1. during mammography.
   2. during fluoroscopy.
   3. during computed tomography.
   4. any time one is in an x-ray room during an examination.
   a. Only 1, 2 and 3 are correct.
   b. Only 1 and 3 are correct.
   c. Only 2 and 4 are correct.
   d. Only 4 is correct.

8. The percentage of all radiographers that receive any measurable occupational radiation exposure each year is approximately
   a. 100.   c. 50.
   b. 75.   d. less than 50.

9. In order to reduce occupational radiation exposure, the following practices are helpful
   1. reducing fluoroscopic examination time
   2. wearing protective apparel during all x-ray examinations
   3. not entering the x-ray room for 5 s after radiography
   4. maintaining as much distance as possible from a fluoroscopic patient
   a. Only 1, 2 and 3 are correct.
   b. Only 1 and 3 are correct.
   c. Only 2 and 4 are correct.
   d. Only 4 is correct.

10. When a single radiation monitor is worn during fluoroscopy, it should be
    a. positioned at waist level under the protective apron.
    b. positioned at waist level outside the protective apron.
    c. clipped to a shirt pocket under the protective apron.
    d. positioned at the collar outside the protective apron.

11. During fluoroscopy the approximate occupational radiation exposure at table side is
    a. 1 mrem/min.   c. 10 mrem/min.
    b. 5 mrem/min.   d. 20 mrem/min.

12. If the only radiographer available to assist during an angiointerventional procedure is 6 weeks pregnant, she should
    a. refuse to do the procedure.
    b. do the procedure observing normal radiation protection practices.
    c. do the procedure because at this time in pregnancy there is little risk.
    d. do the procedure but wear two protective aprons.

13. The approximate annual occupational radiation exposure received by a radiologic technologist is
    a. 5 mrem.   c. 50 mrem.
    b. 10 mrem.   d. 100 mrem.

14. Occupational radiation exposure is lower when
    1. fluoroscopic x-ray beam time is restricted.
    2. a protective apron is worn during fluoroscopy.
    3. the radiologist remains outside the CT examination room.
    4. the radiation monitor is worn under the protective apron.
    a. Only 1, 2 and 3 are correct.
    b. Only 1 and 3 are correct.
    c. Only 2 and 4 are correct.
    d. All are correct.

15. Which of the following is an appropriate radiation protection measure to be implemented **only during pregnancy?**
    1. assign a second occupational radiation monitor
    2. wear two protective aprons
    3. position a second occupational radiation monitor under the protective apron at waist level
    4. undergo no fluoroscopy
    a. Only 1, 2 and 3 are correct.
    b. Only 1 and 3 are correct.
    c. Only 2 and 4 are correct.
    d. All are correct.

16. When a protective apron is worn, it should have a lead equivalency of at least
    a. 0.5 mm.   c. 2 mm.
    b. 1 mm.   d. 4 mm.

17. When a radiologist becomes pregnant, she
    a. should be removed from fluoroscopy.
    b. be given an additional protective apron.
    c. follow normal radiation protection procedures.
    d. institute a set of more restrictive radiation protection procedures.

18. An angiointerventional radiologist averages an estimated 3,000 mrem/y to the lens. What special radiation protection practices are necessary?
    a. reduce workload
    b. wear an additional protective apron
    c. wear protective eye shields
    d. none

19. Occupational radiation exposure is significantly lower when
    1. the radiation monitor is positioned at the collar.
    2. two protective aprons are worn.
    3. a faster image receptor is used for radiography.
    4. the technologist takes one step away from the table during fluoroscopy.

    a. Only 1, 2 and 3 are correct.
    b. Only 1 and 3 are correct.
    c. Only 2 and 4 are correct.
    d. Only 4 is correct.

20. Which of the following is an appropriate radiation protection measure to be implemented **only during pregnancy**?
    1. performing no computed tomography
    2. officially declaring the pregnancy.
    3. positioning a second occupational radiation monitor outside the protective apron at waist level.
    4. color-coding a second occupational radiation monitor so that it is not confused with the collar-positioned monitor.

    a. Only 1, 2, and 3 are correct.
    b. Only 1 and 3 are correct.
    c. Only 2 and 4 are correct.
    d. All are correct.

21. A busy radiologist records 4,500 mrem this year on a collar-positioned radiation monitor. Next year she should
    a. reduce her workload.
    b. wear a thicker protective apron.
    c. wear a protective thyroid collar.
    d. do nothing different.

22. During C-arm fluoroscopy
    a. occupational exposures are highest with the x-ray tube over the patient.
    b. occupational exposures are highest with the x-ray tube under the patient.
    c. a thicker or additional lead apron should be worn.
    d. protective lens and thyroid shields should be worn.

23. During fluoroscopy, the technologist's radiation exposure from scatter radiation 1 m to the side of the patient is approximately what percentage of the patient's exposure?

    a. 0.001   c. 0.1
    b. 0.01   d. 1

24. A protective lead apron attenuates approximately what percentage of scatter radiation?

    a. 1   c. 50
    b. 10   d. 90

25. During portable radiography the proper position for the technologist is

    a. next to the patient.
    b. at the operating console.
    c. 6 ft beyond the operating console.
    d. in the adjacent room.

26. The design of a diagnostic x-ray tube housing must reduce leakage at 1 m to not more than

    a. 1 mR/min.   c. 10 mR/h.
    b. 10 mR/min. d. 100 mR/h.

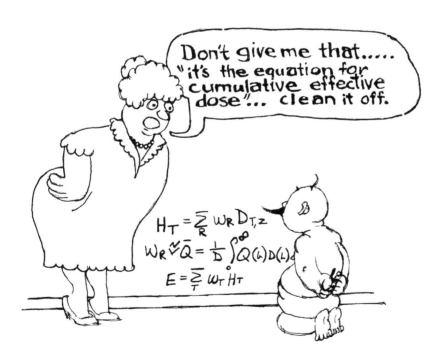

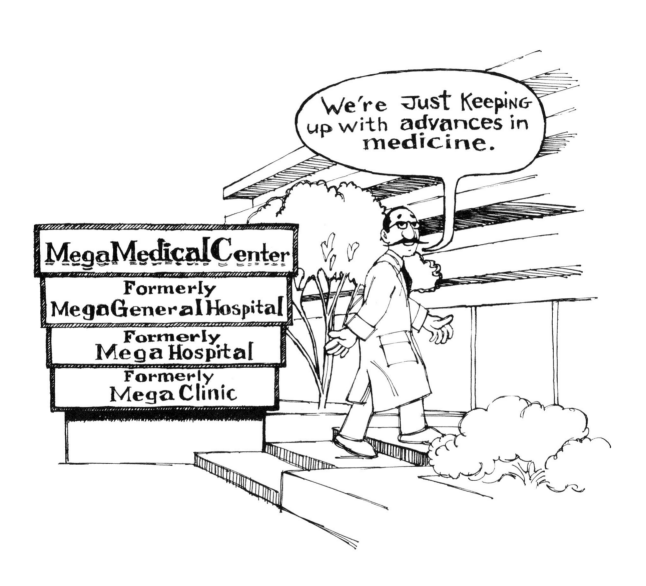

Recommended Radiation Dose Limits

- Radiation dose limits were called **tolerance doses** early in the twentieth century.

- From approximately 1940 to 1990, radiation dose limits were known as **maximum permissible doses (MPD)**.

- Currently occupational radiation dose limits are referred to simply as recommended **dose limits (DL)**.

- Dose limits are recommended for occupational exposure, public exposure, education and training exposure, and exposure of an embryo or fetus.

- In the United States, recommendations for dose limitation are issued by the National Council on Radiation Protection and Measurements (NCRP).

- Recommended dose limits are expressed as **effective dose (E)**.

- Effective dose is measured in rem.

- Recommended dose limits for radiation workers are set at a risk level comparable to that for workers in other industrial occupations.

- Recommended dose limits for the general public are set at a risk level comparable to those experienced by the public under other similar circumstances.

- Recommended dose limits are based on both stochastic and deterministic effects.

- A **stochastic radiation response** is one in which the probability of occurrence increases with increasing effective dose.

- A stochastic radiation response is an all-or-nothing response.

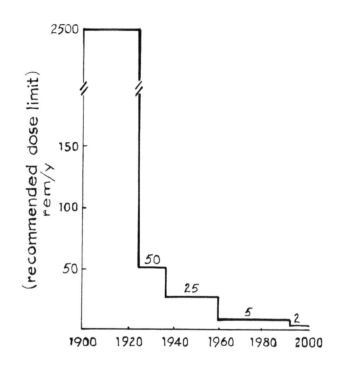

Effective Dose (E) equals the product of Tissue weighting factor (W_T), radiation weighting factor (W_R) and absorbed dose (H_T)

$$E = \sum W_T W_R H_T$$

History of Dose Limitation

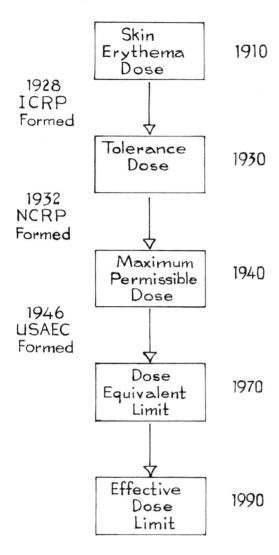

1928
ICRP
Formed

Skin
Erythema
Dose — 1910

Tolerance
Dose — 1930

1932
NCRP
Formed

Maximum
Permissible
Dose — 1940

1946
USAEC
Formed

Dose
Equivalent
Limit — 1970

Effective
Dose
Limit — 1990

Since $W_R = 1$ for X- and γ-rays ....

$$E = \sum W_T H_T$$

- Cancer, leukemia, and genetic effects are the main stochastic radiation responses.

- A **deterministic radiation response** increases in severity with increasing effective dose.

- A deterministic radiation response does not occur below a dose threshold.

- Deterministic late-radiation responses are degenerative, resulting in organ atrophy and fibrosis.

- Much higher radiation doses are required for deterministic responses than for stochastic responses.

- Deterministic radiation responses include skin burns, lens opacification, blood changes, and a decrease in sperm count in the male.

- In medical imaging, deterministic radiation responses are most likely to be observed in patients rather than in radiation workers.

- During x-ray imaging, deterministic radiation effects are most likely to occur during pregnancy or to the skin of angiointerventional patients.

- Recommended dose limits are all below the threshold value for deterministic radiation responses.

- Recommended dose limits are set at a level to limit the risk of stochastic effects to the level of nonradiation risks in society.

- Recommended dose limits are based on the linear, nonthreshold dose-response relationship.

- Regardless of the recommended dose limits, radiation protection practices should be geared to implement ALARA—maintain doses as low as reasonably achievable.

- Recommended dose limits are an acceptable upper limit of exposure, not a design criterion.

- Recommended dose limits are designed to provide radiation protection comparable to that extended to workers in other safe industries.

- Recommended dose limits are based on considerations of accidental death and shortened life span.

- When evaluating shortened life span, fatal accidents result in more lost life expectancy (LLE) than fatal radiogenic cancers.

- Industrial accidents tend to occur in younger males.

Accidental Fatalities in Various Occupations

Occupation	Annual Fatal Accident Rate (per 10,000 workers)
Trade	0.5
Manufacturing	0.6
Service	0.7
Government	0.9
Transportation and utilities	2.7
Construction	3.9
Agriculture	4.6
Mining, quarrying	6.0
All industries (U.S.)	1.1

Source: National Safety Council, *Accident Facts 1994.*

Approximately 1 in 10,000 will die because of

. . . working one year in a safe industry.
. . . receiving 5000 mrem whole body.
. . . smoking 10 packs of cigarettes.
. . . living with a smoker for 15 yrs.
. . . drinking 50 bottles of wine.
. . . a 1000 mile bike ride.
. . . commuting a total of 30,000 miles by car.
. . . 10,000 hr. flying time.
. . . living 15 yrs. in Denver rather than Houston.

- Radiogenic cancer tends to occur in old people.

- According to the National Safety Council, the average annual rate for accidental death in all U.S. industries is approximately 1 in 10,000 workers (10^{-4}).

- Relatively hazardous occupations include agriculture, with five deaths per 10,000 workers annually (5×10^{-4}), and mining, with six deaths per 10,000 workers a year (6×10^{-4}).

- Recommended dose limits are based on safe industries having an annual fatal accident rate of 1 per 10,000 (10^{-4}) or less.

- The risk of dying in an accident while commuting to work by automobile is approximately 1 in 10,000 per year (10^{-4}).

- If one receives the dose limit in a year, the risk of dying from cancer or leukemia later in life is equal to the risk of dying that year in an automobile accident while commuting.

Recommended Values of W_R for Various Types of Radiation

Type of Radiation	Approximate Value of Q
X rays, γ rays, α particles, and electrons	1
Thermal neutrons	5
Neutrons (other than thermal), protons, and α particles	20

Source: National Council on Radiation Protection and Measurements Report 91, 1987.

Tissue Weighting Factors (W_T)

Tissue (T)	W_T
Gonads	0.20
bone marrow	0.12
Colon	0.12
Lungs	0.12
Stomach	0.12
Bladder	0.05
Breasts	0.05
Esophagus	0.05
Liver	0.05
Thyroid	0.05
Bone Surfaces	0.01
Skin	0.01
Remainder	0.05

Recommended Values of the Weighting Factors (W_T) and the Risk Coefficients from Which They Were Derived

Tissue	Risk Coefficient	W_T
Gonads	40×10^{-6} rem^{-1}	0.25
Breast	25×10^{-6} rem^{-1}	0.15
Red bone marrow	20×10^{-6} rem^{-1}	0.12
Lung	20×10^{-6} rem^{-1}	0.12
Thyroid	5×10^{-6} rem^{-1}	0.03
Bone surfaces	5×10^{-6} rem^{-1}	0.03
Remainder	50×10^{-6} rem^{-1}	0.30
Total	165×10^{-6} rem^{-1}	1.00

Source: International Commission on Radiological Protection, Publication 26, 1977.

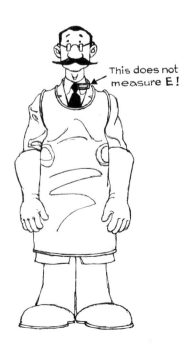

This does not measure E!

- The radiation weighting factor (W_R) is used to weight the relative effectiveness of different types of ionizing radiation.

- The radiation weighting factor is to radiation protection as relative biological effectiveness (RBE) is to radiation biology.

- The radiation weighting factor is principally related to the linear energy transfer (LET) of radiation.

- The radiation weighting factor for diagnostic x-rays is 1.

- The radiation weighting factor for nuclear medicine γ rays is 1.

- Effective dose (E) takes into account the different radiation sensitivity of various tissues and organs.

- E takes into account the different risks of death from cancer in various tissues and organs.

- E takes into account the risk of severe hereditary effects in the first two generations.

- The relative radiosensitivity of tissues and organs is expressed by the tissue weighting factor (W_T).

- The occupational radiation monitor does not measure E; however, for regulatory compliance it is considered to be E.

- The recommended dose limit for occupational exposure is an annual effective dose of 5,000 mrem.

- 5,000 mrem is equal to 5 rem.

- The recommended cumulative dose limit for occupational exposure is 1,000 mrem times the worker's age.

Recommended Dose Limits

Exposure	Dosage
Occupational exposure	
Effective dose equivalent limit (stochastic effects)	5,000 mrem/y
Dose equivalent limits for tissues and organs (deterministic effects)	
Lens of eye	15,000 mrem/y
All others (e.g., red bone marrow, breast, lung, gonads, skin, and extremities)	50,000 mrem/y
Cumulative exposure	1000 mrem x age in years
Public exposure	
Effective dose equivalent limit, continuous exposure	100 mrem/y
Effective dose equivalent limit, infrequent exposure	500 mrem/y
Education and training exposure	
Effective dose equivalent limit related to education and/or training	100 mrem/y
Embryo or fetus exposure	
Total dose equivalent limit	500 mrem
Monthly dose equivalent limit	50 mrem

Source: National Council on Radiation Protection and Measurements Report 91, 1987.

- Dose limits recommended to avoid nonstochastic effects are prescribed for the lens of the eye and for all other tissues or organs individually, including the skin and extremities.

- The annual dose limit for the lens of the eye is 15,000 mrem.

- The annual dose limit for the skin is 50,000 mrem.

- The annual dose limit for the extremities is 50,000 mrem.

- The annual dose limit for individual tissues or organs is 50,000 mrem.

- The annual dose limit for the thyroid is 50,000 mrem.

- A special dose limit is prescribed for protection of the embryo or fetus.

- Mental retardation related to irradiation of the embryo or fetus has been observed only when exposure occurred between weeks 8 and 25 of pregnancy.

- Mental retardation is significant only for irradiation between weeks 8 and 15 of pregnancy.

Occupational Dose Limits

Annual whole body	5000 mrem (50 mSv)
Cumulative whole body	1000 mrem X N (10mSvXN)
Annual, lens	15,000 mrem (150 mSv)
Annual, thyroid	50,000 mrem (500 mSv)
Annual, skin	50,000 mrem (500 mSv)
Annual, extremities	50,000 mrem (500 mSv)

Dose Limit to the Embryo-fetus
of a radiographer/radiologist

50 mrem/mo. (0.5 mSv/mo.)
once declared
500 mrem (5 mSv) Total

Dose Limits to the Public
infrequently exposed   500 mrem/y (5 mSv/y)
frequently exposed   1000 mrem/y (1 mSv/y)
students   100 mrem/y (1 mSv/y)

- The recommended dose limit for the embryo or fetus is 500 mrem.

- Once a pregnancy is known, the recommended dose limit for the embryo or fetus takes precedence over the dose limit for the pregnant radiation worker.

- Once a pregnancy is declared, the recommended dose limit for the embryo or fetus is 50 mrem/month.

- Special dose limits are recommended for members of the public.

- Public radiation dose limits are established to be comparable to other public risks.

- The annual natural background radiation exposure is approximately 100 mrem.

- The lifetime risk from natural background radiation (100 mrem/y) is approximately 1 in 100,000 (10^{-5}).

- The recommended annual dose limit for members of the public who are frequently exposed is 100 mrem.

- The recommended dose limit for members of the public who are rarely exposed is 500 mrem.

- When designing radiation facilities to protect members of the public, one must assume frequent public exposure.

- Persons in training above the age of 18 are subject to the recommended dose limits for occupational exposure.

- Trainees under age 18 are subject to a special recommended dose limit.

- When someone under 18 years of age is engaged in educational or training activities, the recommended dose is 100 mrem/y.

Chapter 8 Practice Questions

1. Which of the following have at some time been used to express recommended radiation dose limits?

   1. tolerance dose
   2. acceptable dose
   3. dose limit
   4. dangerous dose

   a. Only 1, 2 and 3 are correct.
   b. Only 1 and 3 are correct.
   c. Only 2 and 4 are correct.
   d. All are correct.

2. Current dose limits are recommended for which groups of people?

   1. those occupationally exposed
   2. the potentially exposed public
   3. those exposed during the course of education and training
   4. those in utero

   a. Only 1, 2 and 3 are correct.
   b. Only 1 and 3 are correct.
   c. Only 2 and 4 are correct.
   d. All are correct.

3. The radiation weighting factor W_R is best described as

   a. the radiation characteristic used to determine equivalent dose.
   b. having units of keV/μm.
   c. being equal to the RBE.
   d. the radiation characteristic used to determine effective dose.

4. The organization in the United States that is principally responsible for recommending radiation dose limits is the

   a. USNRC.   c. ICRP.
   b. NCRP.   d. USFDA.

5. Recommended dose limits are expressed as

   a. exposure.   c. dose equivalent.
   b. dose.   d. effective dose.

6. Dose equivalent is measured in

   a. R.   c. rem.
   b. rad.   d. Ci.

7. Which of the following best defines effective dose (*E*)?

   a. average equivalent dose to the whole population
   b. equivalent dose responsible for stochastic effects
   c. average equivalent dose to an affected tissue or organ
   d. uniform whole-body equivalent dose expected to produce the same effect as a given partial-body dose

8. When does the equivalent dose equal the effective dose?

   a. when the whole body is irradiated

   b. when the organ of interest is irradiated

   c. when the radiation is delivered acutely

   d. when the biological end point is death

9. Effective dose is measured in

   a. roentgen.   c. rem.

   b. rad.   d. curies.

10. Dose equivalent is measured by which of the following?

   1. roentgen   3. gray

   2. rem   4. sievert

   a. Only 1, 2, and 3 are correct.

   b. Only 1 and 3 are correct.

   c. Only 2 and 4 are correct.

   d. Only 4 is correct.

11. Effective dose can be measured in

   1. roentgen   3. gray

   2. rem   4. sievert

   a. Only 1, 2, and 3 are correct.

   b. Only 1 and 3 are correct.

   c. Only 2 and 4 are correct.

   d. Only 4 is correct.

12. Recommended dose limits for radiation workers are set at a level

   a. considered absolutely safe—zero risk.

   b. at the level of sensitivity of the radiation monitor.

   c. at a risk level comparable to that for other industries.

   d. at a risk level just below the threshold of injury.

13. Recommended dose limits for the general public are set at a risk level

   a. equal to background radiation.

   b. at the sensitivity level of radiation monitors.

   c. at one-tenth the risk level of radiation workers.

   d. comparable to other daily risks.

14. A stochastic radiation response is one

   a. at the recommended dose limit.

   b. where the probability of response increases with increasing dose.

   c. at the threshold dose level.

   d. where the response severity is proportional to dose.

15. Which of the following is considered a stochastic radiation response?

   a. skin erythema   c. cataracts

   b. leukemia   d. moist desquamation

16. Which of the following is considered a stochastic radiation response?
    a. breast cancer
    c. epilation
    b. an x-ray burn
    d. cataracts

17. Recommended dose limits are based
    a. principally on stochastic radiation responses.
    b. principally on deterministic radiation responses.
    c. on both stochastic and deterministic radiation responses.
    d. on neither stochastic nor deterministic radiation responses.

18. A stochastic radiation response is one that
    a. occurs following only low doses.
    b. occurs following only high doses.
    c. follows a threshold-type dose-response relationship.
    d. is an all-or-nothing-type response.

19. Which of the following is considered a stochastic radiation response?
    1. liver cancer
    3. genetic effects
    2. leukemia
    4. skin erythema
    a. Only 1, 2 and 3 are correct.
    b. Only 1 and 3 are correct.
    c. Only 2 and 4 are correct.
    d. All are correct.

20. A deterministic radiation response
    a. has a threshold dose.
    b. exhibits increased incidence with increasing dose.
    c. follows a low radiation dose.
    d. may not be expressed during a lifetime.

21. Deterministic radiation responses
    a. increase in severity with increasing dose.
    b. increase in incidence with increasing dose.
    c. occur at all doses.
    d. include genetic mutations.

22. Which of the following is classified as a deterministic radiation response?
    1. organ atrophy
    3. tissue fibrosis
    2. leukemia
    4. inheritable disease
    a. Only 1, 2, and 3 are correct.
    b. Only 1 and 3 are correct.
    c. Only 2 and 4 are correct.
    d. Only 4 is correct.

23. Which of the following responses require the highest radiation dose?
    a. moist desquamation
    b. leukemia
    c. breast cancer
    d. genetic mutations

24. Which of the following is a deterministic radiation response?
    1. skin erythema   3. hematological depression
    2. lens opacification   4. lowered sperm count
    a. Only 1, 2 and 3 are correct.
    b. Only 1 and 3 are correct.
    c. Only 2 and 4 are correct.
    d. All are correct.

25. Which of the following is a deterministic radiation response?
    1. breast cancer   3. genetic mutations
    2. leukemia   4. moist desquamation
    a. Only 1, 2, and 3 are correct.
    b. Only 1 and 3 are correct.
    c. Only 2 and 4 are correct.
    d. Only 4 is correct.

26. Which of the following is a stochastic radiation response?
    1. skin erythema   3. hematological depression
    2. thyroid cancer   4. genetic mutations
    a. Only 1, 2, and 3 are correct.
    b. Only 1 and 3 are correct.
    c. Only 2 and 4 are correct.
    d. Only 4 is correct.

27. Which of the following is a stochastic radiation response?
    1. skin cancer   3. thyroid cancer
    2. skin erythema   4. epilation
    a. Only 1, 2, and 3 are correct.
    b. Only 1 and 3 are correct.
    c. Only 2 and 4 are correct.
    d. All are correct.

28. Which of the following are more likely to experience a deterministic response?
    1. an angiointerventional patient
    2. a radiographer
    3. an angiographer
    4. an ultrasound technologist
    a. Only 1, 2, and 3 are correct.
    b. Only 1 and 3 are correct.
    c. Only 2 and 4 are correct.
    d. Only 4 is correct.

29. Recommended dose limits are below the
    a. threshold for deterministic responses.
    b. threshold for stochastic responses.
    c. threshold of the radiation monitor.
    d. sensitivity of the radiation monitor.

30. Recommended dose limits are based on which type of radiation dose-response relationship?

    a. linear, threshold
    b. linear, nonthreshold
    c. nonlinear, threshold
    d. nonlinear, nonthreshold

31. The term ALARA refers to

    1. using low-mA or -mAs technique.
    2. using low-kVp technique.
    3. care in patient selection.
    4. minimizing radiation exposure.

    a. Only 1, 2, and 3 are correct.
    b. Only 1 and 3 are correct.
    c. Only 2 and 4 are correct.
    d. Only 4 is correct.

32. The practice of ALARA in medical imaging refers to

    a. at last a recommended average.
    b. at last a rational action.
    c. a level at reasonable action.
    d. as low as reasonably achievable.

33. Recommended dose limits for workers are set comparable to risk to those for

    a. the general public.
    b. workers in safe industries.
    c. workers in all industries.
    d. workers in hazardous industries.

34. When establishing recommended dose limits, which of the following is considered?

    a. type of industry
    b. accidental death rate
    c. occupational classification
    d. gender of the worker

35. When establishing recommended dose limits, which of the following are considered?

    a. average age of the population
    b. expected number of children of the worker
    c. severity of disease
    d. lost life expectancy

36. Which of the following is expected to result in the most lost life expectancy?

    a. automobile accidents
    b. breast cancer
    c. prostate cancer
    d. genetic mutations

37. Accidents in hazardous industries tend to occur among
    a. younger females.   c. younger males
    b. older females.   d. older males.

38. Radiation-induced cancer tends to occur in
    1. younger females.   3. younger males.
    2. older females.   4. older males.
    a. Only 1, 2 and 3 are correct.
    b. Only 1 and 3 are correct.
    c. Only 2 and 4 are correct.
    d. Only 4 is correct.

39. The average annual accidental death rate in U.S. industry is
    a. 1 in 1,000 (10^{-3}).   c. 1 in 100,000 (10^{-5}).
    b. 1 in 10,000 (10^{-4}).   d. 1 in 1 million (10^{-6}).

40. The average annual accidental death rate in the most hazardous industries is closest to
    a. 1 in 1,000 (10^{-3}).   c. 1 in 100,000 (10^{-5}).
    b. 1 in 10,000 (10^{-4}).   d. 1 in 1 million (10^{-6}).

41. The risk of dying in an acccident while commuting to work by automobile is approximately
    a. 1 in 1,000 (10^{-3}).   c. 1 in 100,000 (10^{-5}).
    b. 1 in 10,000 (10^{-4}).   d. 1 in 1 million (10^{-6}).

42. If you receive an occupational effective dose of 1,000 mrem this year, your risk of dying later in life because of that exposure is closest to
    a. 1 in 1,000 (10^{-3}).   c. 1 in 100,000 (10^{-5}).
    b. 1 in 10,000 (10^{-4}).   d. 1 in 1 million (10^{-6}).

43. The term **quality factor** (Q)
    a. varies with different radiations.
    b. varies for different tissue.
    c. varies as a function of age and gender.
    d. is measured in rem.

44. Quality factor is most analogous to
    a. linear energy transfer (LET).
    b. effective dose equivalent (H_E).
    c. absorbed dose (D).
    d. relative biological effectiveness (RBE).

45. Dose equivalent (H_E) is
    a. the product of absorbed dose (D) and linear energy transfer (LET).
    b. the product of absorbed dose (D) and quality factor (Q).
    c. the sum of absorbed dose (D) and quality factor (Q).
    d. the sum of quality factor (Q) and linear energy transfer (LET).

46. Dose equivalent

    1. can be measured in rem.
    2. can be measured in sievert.
    3. is the product of absorbed dose (D) and quality factor (Q).
    4. is the sum of quality factor (Q) and linear energy transfer (LET).

    a. Only 1, 2 and 3 are correct.
    b. Only 1 and 3 are correct.
    c. Only 2 and 4 are correct.
    d. All are correct.

47. Quality factor is principally related to

    a. RBE.
    b. OER.
    c. H_E.
    d. LET.

48. The quality factor for diagnostic x-rays is approximately

    a. 0.3.
    b. 1.0.
    c. 3.0.
    d. 10.0.

49. The quality factor for nuclear medicine γ rays is approximately

    a. 0.3.
    b. 1.0.
    c. 3.0.
    d. 10.0.

50. Recommended dose limits

    a. are expressed in rad.
    b. are expressed in rem.
    c. vary for different types of radiation.
    d. vary for different occupations.

51. Recommended dose limits are

    a. expressed in gray.
    b. expressed in rad.
    c. expressed as dose equivalent (H).
    d. expressed as effective dose (E).

52. Effective dose takes into account

    a. the gender of the worker.
    b. the occupation of the worker.
    c. the risk of various types of accidental deaths.
    d. the radiogenic sensitivity of various tissues.

53. Effective dose accounts for

    1. type of accident.
    2. severe hereditary effects.
    3. congenital abnormalities.
    4. various tissue radiosensitivity.

    a. Only 1, 2 and 3 are correct.
    b. Only 1 and 3 are correct.
    c. Only 2 and 4 are correct.
    d. Only 4 is correct.

54. The relative radiosensitivity of tissues and organs is represented by
    a. relative biological effectiveness (RBE).
    b. weighting factor (W_T).
    c. as low as reasonably achievable (ALARA).
    d. quality factor (Q).

55. The recommended annual dose limit for a radiation worker is
    a. a whole-body dose of 5,000 mrem.
    b. an effective dose equivalent of 5,000 mrem.
    c. a whole-body dose of 500 mrem.
    d. an effective dose equivalent of 500 mrem.

56. Last year you received an effective dose of 650 mrem. How many rem is this?
    a. 0.065 rem   c. 6.5 rem
    b. 0.650 rem   d. 65 rem

57. Your monthly film badge report shows an effective dose of 50 mrem. This is equivalent to
    a. 0.005 rem.   c. 0.5 rem.
    b. 0.05 rem.   d. 5 rem.

58. Which of the following is the recommended cumulative dose limit for a radiographer or radiologist?
    1. 5,000 mrem times age
    2. 1,000 mrem times age
    3. 5 rem times age
    4. 1 rem times age

    a. Only 1, 2 and 3 are correct.
    b. Only 1 and 3 are correct.
    c. Only 2 and 4 are correct.
    d. Only 4 is correct.

59. If N = a radiation worker's age, which of the following expresses the cumulative dose limit?
    a. 1,000 mrem $\times$ N
    b. 5,000 mrem $\times$ N
    c. 1,000 mrem $\times$ (N − 18)
    d. 5,000 mrem $\times$ (N − 18)

60. If N = a radiation worker's age, which of the following expresses the cumulative dose limit?
    a. 10 mSv $\times$ N c. 10 mSv $\times$ (N − 18)
    b. 50 mSv $\times$ N d. 50 mSv $\times$ (N − 18)

61. The recommended dose limit established for the lens of the eye is based principally on
    a. stochastic effects.
    b. deterministic effects.
    c. age-related effects.
    d. gender-related effects.

62. The recommended dose limit established for the thyroid is based principally on

    a. stochastic effects.
    b. deterministic effects.
    c. age-related effects.
    d. gender-related effects.

63. The recommended dose limit established for the skin is based principally on

    a. stochastic effects.
    b. deterministic effects.
    c. age-related effects.
    d. gender-related effects.

64. The recommended dose limit established for the extremities is based principally on

    a. stochastic effects.
    b. deterministic effects.
    c. age-related effects.
    d. gender-related effects.

65. Consideration of stochastic radiation responses is used in establishing

    1. annual occupational dose limits.
    2. dose limits to the extremities.
    3. cumulative occupational dose limits.
    4. dose limits to the thyroid.

    a. Only 1, 2 and, 3 are correct.
    b. Only 1 and 3 are correct.
    c. Only 2 and 4 are correct.
    d. All are correct.

66. Deterministic radiation responses are used in establishing

    1. annual occupational dose limits.
    2. dose limits to the extremities.
    3. cumulative occupational dose limits.
    4. dose limits to the lens.

    a. Only 1, 2, and 3 are correct.
    b. Only 1 and 3 are correct.
    c. Only 2 and 4 are correct.
    d. Only 4 is correct.

67. The annual dose limit for the lens of the eye is

    a. 500 mrem.   c. 5,000 mrem.
    b. 1,500 mrem.   d. 15,000 mrem.

68. The annual dose limit for the skin is

    a. 500 mrem.   c. 15,000 mrem.
    b. 5,000 mrem.   d. 50,000 mrem.

69. The annual dose limit for the upper extremities is

    a. 1,000 mrem.   c. 15,000 mrem.
    b. 5,000 mrem.   d. 50,000 mrem.

70. The annual dose limit for the lower extremities is
    a. 1,000 mrem.   c. 15,000 mrem.
    b. 5,000 mrem.   d. 50,000 mrem.

71. The annual dose limit for the thyroid is
    a. 1,000 mrem.   c. 15,000 mrem.
    b. 5,000 mrem.   d. 50,000 mrem.

72. One of the suspected responses following irradiation in utero is
    a. sex change.   c. extended pregnancy.
    b. premature birth.   d. mental retardation.

73. Suspected mental retardation following irradiation in utero is significant when it occurs
    a. any time during pregnancy.
    b. between the eighth and fifteenth weeks of pregnancy.
    c. between the fifteenth and twenty-fifth weeks of pregnancy.
    d. after the twenty-fifth week of pregnancy.

74. Exposure to radiation during pregnancy can produce which of the following suspected responses?
    1. mental retardation   3. stunted growth
    2. childhood cancer   4. congenital abnormalities

    a. Only 1, 2, and 3 are correct.
    b. Only 1 and 3 are correct.
    c. Only 2 and 4 are correct.
    d. All are correct.

75. Once a pregnancy is known,
    a. a radiation worker should cease radiation work.
    b. a member of the public should not enter a radiation area.
    c. the embryo or fetus dose limit takes precedence over the public dose limit.
    d. the embryo or fetus dose limit takes precedence over the radiation worker dose limit.

76. Once a pregnancy is known,
    1. a radiologist should perform no fluoroscopy.
    2. the radiographer's dose limit is reduced.
    3. special protective apparel is required for workers and patients.
    4. the embryo or fetus dose limit is lower than that for the radiologist.

    a. Only 1, 2 and 3 are correct.
    b. Only 1 and 3 are correct.
    c. Only 2 and 4 are correct.
    d. Only 4 is correct.

77. Once a pregnancy is declared,
    1. the radiologist should perform no more fluoroscopy.
    2. the radiographer's dose limit is reduced.
    3. special protective apparel should be obtained.
    4. an additional radiation monitor should be obtained.

a. Only 1, 2 and 3 are correct.
b. Only 1 and 3 are correct.
c. Only 2 and 4 are correct.
d. Only 4 is correct.

78. Once a pregnancy is declared, the recommended dose limit for the

a. embryo or fetus is 50 mrem/month.
b. embryo or fetus is 500 mrem/month.
c. radiologist is 500 mrem/month.
d. radiologist is 5,000 mrem/month.

79. Once a pregnancy is declared, the recommended dose limit for the embryo or fetus is

a. 50 mrem/month.
b. 50 mrem/9 months.
c. 500 mrem/y.
d. 5000 mrem/y.

80. The annual dose limit of 100 mrem applies to

1. natural background radiation.
2. the embryo or fetus.
3. the infrequently exposed public.
4. the frequently exposed public.

a. Only 1, 2 and 3 are correct.
b. Only 1 and 3 are correct.
c. Only 2 and 4 are correct.
d. Only 4 is correct.

81. The lifetime risk from annual exposure to natural background radiation is estimated to be approximately

a. 1 in 1000 (10^{-3}).   c. 1 in 100,000 (10^{-5}).
b. 1 in 10,000 (10^{-4}).   d. 1 in 1 million (10^{-6}).

82. Which of the following is associated with a dose of 500 mrem?

1. dose limit to the embryo or fetus
2. dose limit for a radiologist during pregnancy
3. annual dose limit for the infrequently exposed public
4. annual dose limit for the frequently exposed public

a. Only 1, 2, and 3 are correct.
b. Only 1 and 3 are correct.
c. Only 2 and 4 are correct.
d. Only 4 is correct.

83. The recommended dose limit for frequently exposed members of the public is

a. 50 mrem/month.   c. 100 mrem/month.
b. 50 mrem/y.   d. 100 mrem/y.

84. The recommended dose limit for members of the public who are not frequently exposed is

a. 50 mrem/month.   c. 50 mrem/y.
b. 500 mrem/month.   d. 500 mrem/y.

85. You are a 17-year-old student radiographer. What is your annual dose limit?

    a. 50 mrem   c. 500 mrem
    b. 100 mrem   d. 5,000 mrem

86. Which of the following is assigned an annual dose limit of 100 mrem?

    1. pregnant radiologists
    2. frequently exposed members of the public
    3. infrequently exposed member of the public
    4. students

    a. Only 1, 2, and 3 are correct.
    b. Only 1 and 3 are correct.
    c. Only 2 and 4 are correct.
    d. Only 4 is correct.

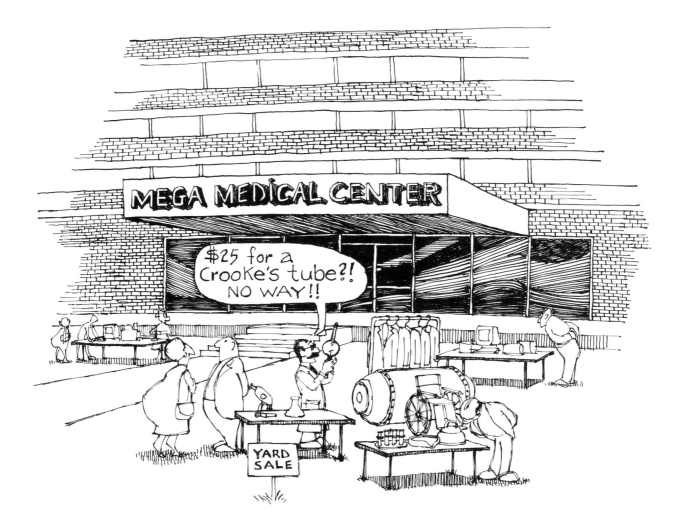

Specialty Areas of Medical Imaging

NUCLEAR MEDICINE IMAGING

- γ rays are used to form images in nuclear medicine.

- γ rays are emitted by radioactive atoms called **radioisotopes**.

- There are two principal hazards in nuclear medicine imaging—contamination and radiation exposure.

- Contamination is the uncontrolled spread of radioactive material.

- Contamination is hazardous because radioactive material can be inhaled or ingested.

- Contamination does not normally present an external radiation hazard.

- Some radioactive sources used in nuclear medicine pose an external radiation hazard.

- Contamination control requires protective clothing such as disposable gloves, gowns, and shoe covers.

- Radioactive contamination has one advantage over biological contamination—small quantities are easily detected.

- Contamination control requires periodic surveys with a Geiger counter or a portable scintillation counter.

- Frequent wipe tests of surfaces are necessary for contamination control.

- Plastic-backed absorbent paper, when placed on work surfaces, helps control radioactive contamination in nuclear medicine laboratories.

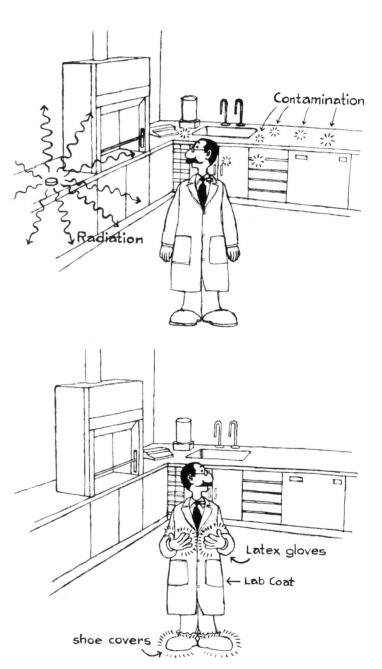

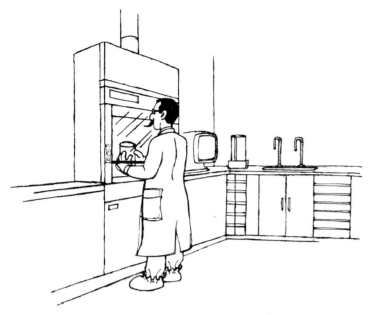

Fume Hood

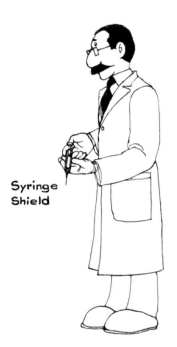

**Syringe
Shield**

Misadministration
- wrong radioisotope
- wrong quantity
- wrong route

- A chemical fume hood without a charcoal filter is required for storage and use of radioactive gases such as ^{131}I and ^{133}Xe.

- Ingestion is minimized by frequent hand washing with soap and warm water.

- No eating, drinking, or smoking should be allowed in radioactive materials areas.

- Wipe tests should be performed daily in a hot laboratory and at least weekly in an imaging laboratory.

- All potentially contaminated items and radioactive waste should be disposed of in designated receptacles.

- When performing ^{133}Xe ventilation studies, the imaging laboratory must be at negative pressure.

- Never pipet radioactive materials by mouth.

- Use syringe and vial shields when handling radioactive material.

- In case of an accident, administer first aid, then decontaminate personnel, and then decontaminate the facility.

- In case of an accident, facility decontamination should begin at the perimeter of the area of and then work toward the center.

- If internal contamination is possible, bioassay may be necessary.

- Monitoring with a scintillation crystal is an acceptable thyroid bioassay procedure.

- Liquid scintillation counting of urine samples is an acceptable bioassay procedure.

- Patient misadministration can be avoided by implementing strict procedures.

- Physician orders must be verified.

- Mode of administration must be verified.

- Quantity of radioactive material must be verified.

- Quantity of radioactive material should be assayed in a dose calibrator.

- Type of radioactive material must be verified.

- Patient misadministration includes using (1) wrong radioisotope, (2) wrong quantity, and (3) wrong mode of administration.

- Nursing mothers should cease breast feeding for at least 24 hours following a ^{99m}Tc diagnostic study.

- Radionuclide therapy with ^{131}I presents special radiation protection problems.

- ^{131}I in capsule form is preferred to that in liquid form.

- ^{131}I is secreted in urine, saliva, and perspiration.

- During ^{131}I therapy the floor of a patient's room must be covered with plastic-backed absorbent paper to prevent contamination.

- ^{131}I therapy patients should be given only disposable utensils.

- Clothes, linens, and towels of ^{131}I therapy patients must be stored for decay before disposal or recycling.

- ^{131}I therapy patients should not be discharged from the hospital until their internal contamination is less than 30 mCi or the exposure rate at 1 m from the patient is less than 5 mR/h.

Dose Calibrator QC	Frequency	if < 10% change
Constancy	Daily	repair or replace
Linearity	Quarterly	correction required
Accuracy	Annually	repair or replace
Geometry	At Installation	correction required

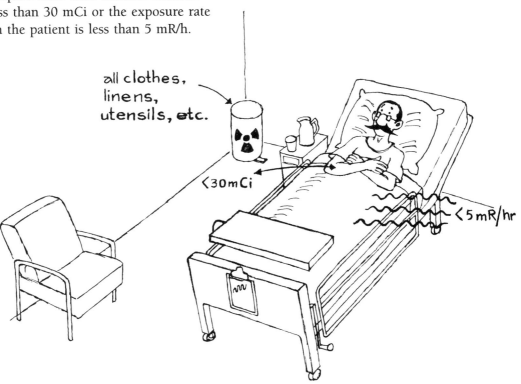

- Generally, nuclear medicine technologists receive lower occupational exposures than radiographers.

- Nuclear medicine technologists should prepare millicurie quantities of radioactive behind protective barriers.

- Nuclear medicine technologists should always employ syringe and vial shields.

- Nuclear medicine technologists should be provided with a ring badge for hand monitoring in addition to a body badge.

- Radioactive waste should be segregated into short-lived and long-lived material.

- Short-lived radioactive waste includes that containing ^{99m}Tc and ^{123}I.

- Long-lived radioactive waste includes that containing ^{67}Ga, ^{131}I, and ^{111}I.

- Radioactive waste should be stored for decay before disposal in the normal solid waste system.

- Before depositing radioactive waste in a storage decay receptacle, remove or obliterate all radiation symbols.

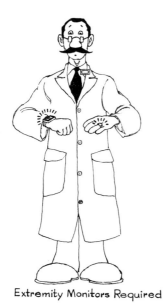

Extremity Monitors Required

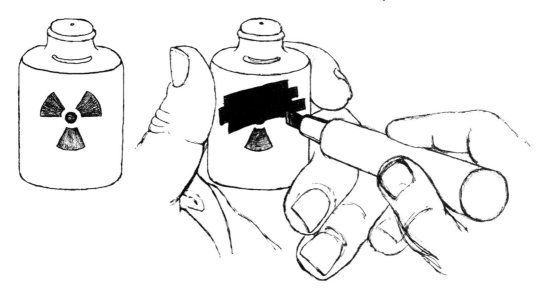

- Radioactive waste must be stored for decay to the level of natural background before disposal in a sanitary waste system.

- Radioactive material used in nuclear medicine is regulated by either the U.S. Nuclear Regulatory Commission (USNRC) or various state health departments.

- State health departments that regulate radio-active material are in agreement states.

- **Agreements states** are those permitted by the USNRC to perform the function of radiation control in that state.

DIAGNOSTIC ULTRASOUND IMAGING

- There are two types of responses to ultrasound exposure—thermal responses and nonthermal responses.

- Both thermal and nonthermal responses have been observed only at intensities much higher than that employed in diagnostic ultrasound.

- Thermal responses are **heating** of soft tissue and bone.

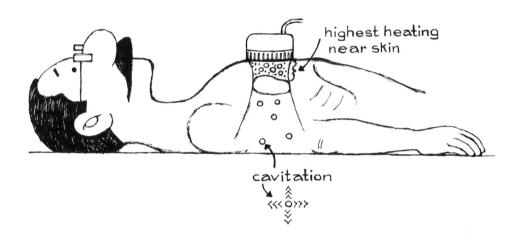

- Nonthermal responses are mechanical in nature—**cavitation, tiny bubble formation,** and **membrane shearing**.

- There has never been a report of patient injury from diagnostic ultrasound examination.

- There are no concerns of operator safety in applications of diagnostic ultrasound.

- There are concerns of patient safety in diagnostic ultrasound because of expanding application and increasing beam intensity.

- For most ultrasound beams, the highest tissue heating occurs near the skin.

- For focused ultrasound beams, the highest temperature tissue heating occurs away from the skin but before the focal region.

Tissue heating f (TA)
mW/cm²

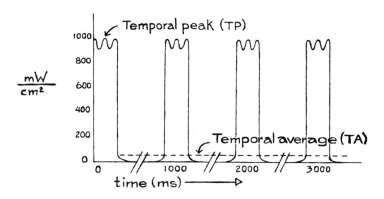

attenuation

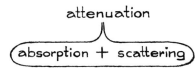

absorption = energy converted to heat
scattering = change in ultrasound direction

- For diagnostic ultrasound beams with long focal lengths, maximum tissue temperature rise occurs closer to the surface.

- For diagnostic ultrasound beams with short focal lengths, maximum tissue heating occurs closer to the focus.

- Biological effects are a function of ultrasound intensity.

- Ultrasound intensity is ultrasound power divided by beam area (mW/cm²).

- Tissue heating by diagnostic ultrasound is principally a function of the temporal average (TA) intensity rather than the temporal peak (TP) intensity.

- TP intensity may be a thousand times higher than TA intensity.

- More important to tissue heating than TA intensity is the time the ultrasonographer fixes the beam on one tissue area.

- Tissue heating results from absorption of energy from the ultrasound beam.

- **Attenuation** of the ultrasound beam is a reduction in intensity with penetration into tissue.

- Ultrasound attenuation has two components (1) energy **absorption** and conversion to heat, and (2) redirection of the beam by **scattering**.

- Tissue heating is also dependent on an ultrasound absorption characteristic called the **absorption coefficient**.

- The ultrasound absorption coefficient is measured in dB/cm/MHz.

- Water in biological fluids has a low ultrasound absorption coefficient.

- Fetal bone and adult bone have a high ultrasound absorption coefficient.

- Soft tissues, skin, and cartilage have intermediate absorption coefficients.

- Tissues with a low absorption coefficient absorb little energy and do not heat.

- Tissues with a high absorption coefficient absorb lots of energy and may experience a temperature rise.

- The higher the ultrasound frequency, the higher the energy absorption.

- The higher the ultrasound frequency, the less the penetration into tissue.

- The principal tissue of concern in diagnostic ultrasound imaging is **fetal bone**.

- Tissue heating is usually considered for three types of tissues—soft tissue, layered tissue, and bone.

- For the examination of homogeneous soft tissue, such as the abdomen, tissue heating is approximately uniform up to the focal length and then decreases rapidly.

- For examination of layered tissue such as a fluid-filled bladder, there is little heating through the bladder and increased heating in the soft tissue at greater depths.

- If bone, especially fetal bone, exists at a depth, tissue heating will be highest at that depth.

- Nonthermal ultrasound responses are not as well understood as thermal ultrasound responses.

- Nonthermal ultrasound responses require higher intensity than thermal ultrasound responses.

- The principal nonthermal response to ultrasound is **cavitation**.

- Cavitation is somewhat related to the spatial peak (SP) intensity of the ultrasound beam.

- Cavitation is not possible at the diagnostic ultrasound intensities currently employed.

- Cavitation has never been observed in an ultrasound patient.

- Since there are no known current risks, the benefit/risk ratio of diagnostic ultrasound is enormous.

- Newer applications and higher possible intensities of diagnostic ultrasound require that it be used with prudence.

- ALARA is a principle that also applies to diagnostic ultrasound.

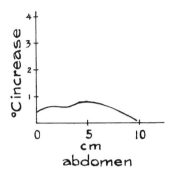

Tissue Heating
6 cm focus

abdomen

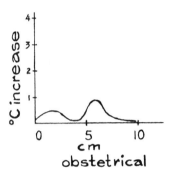

obstetrical

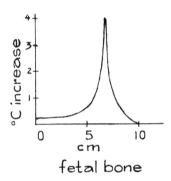

fetal bone

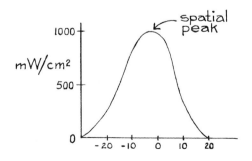

- ALARA in diagnostic ultrasound is applied by maintaining a low output intensity when possible.

- ALARA requires an ultrasonographer to select the lowest output intensity consistent with good image quality.

- ALARA is implemented by an ultrasonographer by selecting the lowest pulse repetition frequency (PRF) consistent with good image quality.

- To implement ALARA, the ultrasonographer should select an intensity-focal depth combination to allow viewing of the anatomy of interest and no deeper.

- To implement ALARA, an ultrasonographer should select the shortest pulse length (PL) consistent with good image quality.

- To implement ALARA, an ultrasonographer should select the lowest frequency transducer consistent with the depth of tissue to be imaged and good image quality.

- Whenever possible, an ultrasonographer should increase receiver gain or time gain control rather than increasing beam intensity.

- An ultrasonographer can reduce patient exposure by minimizing scan time and performing only the required scans.

- An ultrasonographer should never rush through an examination because a reexamination may then be necessary.

- The newest ultrasound imagers have three meters each of which registers a scanning index on a scale of 1 to 4 to help the ultrasonographer maintain exposure ALARA.

- The **mechanical index (MI)** indicates the potential for nonthermal effects.

- The **soft tissue thermal index (TIS)** is related to temperature increases within soft homogeneous tissues.

- The **cranial bone thermal index (TIC)** is related to potential temperature increase in bone at or near the surface such as during a cranial examination.

- The **bone thermal index (TIB)** is helpful in maintaining fetal bone exposure ALARA.

To implement ALARA,
use minimal:
PRF
PL
scan time
MI
TIS
TIC
TIB

- The numerical value of the scanning index is related to relative tissue heating but not to an actual value of temperature.

- In order to implement ALARA, the ultrasonographer should keep the scanning index as low as possible, as well as the examination time.

- Nuclear medicine patients referred for ultrasonography are not a radiation hazard to the ultrasonographer.

MAGNETIC RESONANCE IMAGING

Three energy fields

- Magnetic resonance images are made with radio waves usually identified as **radio frequency (RF)**.

- RF is electromagnetic radiation positioned at the long-wavelength end of the electromagnetic spectrum.

- RF has relatively low energy and relatively low frequency.

- The RF employed for magnetic resonance imaging (MRI) ranges from approximately 10 to 100 MHz.

- The intensity of the RF field is expressed as **specific absorption rate (SAR)** in watts per kilogram (W/kg).

- There are two energy fields involved in MRI in addition to RF—the **primary magnetic field** B_0 and the **gradient magnetic fields** B_{xyz}.

- The B_0 field is measured in tesla (T).

- The B_0 field has constant intensity.

- The gradient magnetic fields are measured in tesla per second (T/s).

- The gradient magnetic fields are termed **transient magnetic fields** because they vary in intensity with time.

MRI Field	units
radiofrequency (RF)	MHz
gradient (Bx,y,z)	T/s
primary (Bo)	T

Interaction with the three energy fields

- The interaction between RF and tissue is thermal.

- Like a microwave oven, sufficiently intense RF can raise the temperature of tissue.

MRI Field	Patient Response
RF	Tissue heating
$B_{x,y,z}$	nerve stimulation
B_o	polarization projectiles

- Several W/kg are required to raise the temperature of soft tissue 1°C.

- A RF-induced temperature rise is dependent on tissue vascularity and time of exposure.

- Heating of avascular tissues such as the lens of the eye can produce cataracts.

- The interaction between the B_0 field and tissue is called **polarization**.

- When tissue is polarized, some of its molecules become aligned with a north and a south pole.

- Tissue polarization is extremely small and disappears when a patient is removed from the magnet.

- The gradient magnetic field interacts with tissue by inducing electric currents when a gradient is being switched on or off and its intensity is rising or falling, respectively.

- When switched on or off, gradient magnetic fields may induce electric currents in central nervous system cells and neurons, stimulating neuronal conduction.

- Sensory nerve stimulation and peripheral nerve stimulation are potential effects of gradient magnetic fields.

- **Magnetophosphenes** (retinal flashes) and a metallic taste in the mouth have been reported by some magnetic resonance imaging (MRI) patients.

- Twitching or tingling in the extremities also has been reported by some MRI patients.

- Ventricular fibrillation is a potential response to the B_{xyz} fields.

- The threshold for ventricular fibrillation is a current density of approximately 0.1 mA/cm^2.

- Clearly the greatest hazard associated with MRI involves the mechanical force exerted on ferromagnetic objects by the B_0 field.

- Projectiles in the imaging room have been reported as causing injury in a few cases.

- A small number of interstitial implants, such as surgical aneurysm clips, have been reported to twist in a patient while aligning with the B_0 field.

MRI intensity limitations

- The U.S. Food and Drug Administration (USFDA) is the agency responsible for MRI patient and personnel protection.

- For clinical imaging, the B_0 field intensity is limited to 2 T.

- For clinical imaging, the B_{xyz} field intensity is limited to 20 T/s.

- For clinical imaging, the RF intensity is limited to 2 W/kg averaged over the entire body or 4 W/g for any 1 g of tissue.

- There are no restrictions on the limit of exposure to these fields for medical personnel.

- Access to MRI by the public is restricted because of concern for the interaction between the fringe magnetic field created by B_0 and cardiac pacemakers.

- Public access to MRI must be restricted so that the fringe magnetic field is less than 0.5 mT (5 G).

- MRI fields all exhibit a threshold intensity-response relationship.

- MRI fields exhibit a nonlinear intensity-response relationship.

- Interference with the completion of a MRI examination occurs in approximately 5% of patients because of claustrophobia.

- Toxic reaction to some contrast enhancement agents has been reported in a vanishingly small number of patients.

- **Pregnancy** is not a contraindication for performing an MRI examination.

- Restrictions on pregnant operators of magnetic resonance imagers are unnecessary.

MRI Field	clinical limitation
RF	4 W/gm or 2 W/kg avg.
$B_{x,y,z}$	20 T/s
B_0	2 T

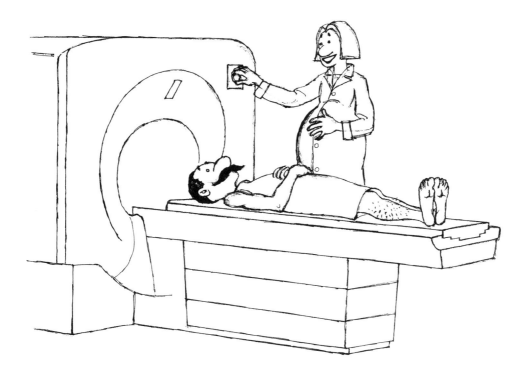

Chapter 9 Practice Questions (Nuclear Medicine Imaging)

1. Which of the following radiations is most useful in nuclear medicine imaging?

   a. α particles   c. γ rays
   b. β particles   d. x rays

2. Which of the following is most helpful in controlling radioactive contamination?

   a. a scintillation detector
   b. a phosphorescent detector
   c. a film badge
   d. an electroscope

3. When imaging with volatile radioactive material,

   a. wipe tests must be performed immediately afterward.
   b. the patient must be provided a radiation dosimeter.
   c. the laboratory should be at negative atmospheric pressure.
   d. the laboratory should be at positive atmospheric pressure.

4. The preferred form of a therapeutic dose of ^{131}I is

   a. hermetically sealed.
   b. a gelatin capsule.
   c. liquid.
   d. gas.

5. Effective radioactive waste disposal includes

    a. monitoring service personnel with a film badge.
    b. obliterating all radioactive symbols before disposal.
    c. segregating radioactive waste by form (liquid-solid).
    d. disposal on the day of generation.

6. Radioisotopes are atoms having the same number of

    a. α particles.   c. protons.
    b. β particles.   d. neutrons.

7. Which of the following is helpful in controlling radioactive contamination?

    1. a Geiger counter
    2. an ionization chamber
    3. periodic wipe tests
    4. personnel monitoring

    a. Only 1, 2, and 3 are correct.
    b. Only 1 and 3 are correct.
    c. Only 2 and 4 are correct.
    d. All are correct.

8. Which of the following are routine radiation protection practices in a nuclear medicine laboratory?

    1. using only automatic pipets
    2. using lead syringe shields
    3. providing a whole-body monitor
    4. providing an extremity radiation monitor

    a. Only 1, 2, and 3 are correct.
    b. Only 1 and 3 are correct.
    c. Only 2 and 4 are correct.
    d. All are correct.

9. Which of the following is appropriate when dealing with an ^{131}I therapy patient?

    a using only disposable utensils
    b. providing the patient with a film badge
    c. daily disposal of linens, etc.
    d. retaining urine and feces for decay

10. The principal agency responsible for the regulation of radioactive material is the

    a. U.S. Nuclear Regulatory Commission.
    b. U.S. Food and Drug Administration.
    c. U.S. Department of Energy.
    d. U.S. Public Health Service.

11. Which of the following are potential hazards in a nuclear medicine laboratory?

    1. radiation exposure
    2. radio-frequency exposure
    3. radioactive contamination
    4. ultrasound contamination

    a. Only 1, 2, and 3 are correct.
    b. Only 1 and 3 are correct.
    c. Only 2 and 4 are correct.
    d. All are correct.

12. a chemical fume hood is necessary in a nuclear medicine laboratory to contain which of the following volatile radioactive gasses?

1. ^{99m}Tc   3. ^{90}Sr

2. ^{131}I   4. ^{133}Xe

   a. Only 1, 2, and 3 are correct.

   b. Only 1 and 3 are correct.

   c. Only 2 and 4 are correct.

   d. All are correct.

13. If a radioactive contamination incident occurs, the following should be done in what order?

   1. apply first aid if necessary

   2. decontaminate personnel

   3. decontaminate the laboratory

   4. notify the radiation safety officer

   a. 1, 2, 3, 4   c. 2, 4, 1, 3

   b. 1, 3, 2, 4   d. 3, 4, 1, 2

14. Discharge of patients undergoing radionuclide therapy must wait until the internal burden of radioactive material is less than

   a. 5 mCi.   c. 20 mCi.

   b. 10 mCi.   d. 30 mCi.

15. Radioactive contamination is

   a. usually measured in mrad.

   b. usually measured in mrem.

   c. encapsulated material.

   d. loose radioactive material.

16. Chemical fume hoods are required in all nuclear medicine laboratories

   a. that employ sealed sources of radioactive material.

   b. for gaseous equipment storage.

   c. for storage of volatile radioisotopes.

   d. for manipulating millicurie quantities of radioactive material.

17. Thyroid monitoring of nuclear medicine personnel is best done with

   a. an ionization chamber.

   b. a scintillation detector.

   c. a film badge.

   d. thermoluminescent dosimeters.

18. Radionuclide therapy patients should not be discharged from the hospital until the exposure rate 1 m from the patient is less than

   a. 1 mR/h.   c. 5 mR/h.

   b. 2 mR/h.   d. 25 mR/h.

19. Radioactive contamination is a potential hazard principally because

   a. the material can be inhaled or ingested.

   b. the resulting exposure can be quite high.

   c. it can be transferred from person to person.

   d. it cannot be easily removed.

20. Which of the following should be prohibited in a nuclear medicine laboratory?

    1. eating   3. drinking
    2. smoking   4. loitering

    a. Only 1, 2, and 3 are correct.
    b. Only 1 and 3 are correct.
    c. Only 2 and 4 are correct.
    d. All are correct.

21. Urinalysis to detect radioactive contamination is best performed with a

    a. crystal scintillation detector.
    b. liquid scintillation detector.
    c. film badge.
    d. thermoluminescent dosimeter.

22. Effective disposal of radioactive waste includes

    a. film badge monitoring.
    b. radiation monitoring of all personnel.
    c. segregation of waste by form.
    d. segregation of waste by half-life.

23. Effective control of radioactive material may involve disposable

    1. gloves.   3. gowns.
    2. shoe covers.   4. countertop mats.

    a. Only 1, 2, and 3 are correct.
    b. Only 1 and 3 are correct.
    c. Only 2 and 4 are correct.
    d. All are correct.

24. The recommended frequency of wipe tests in a hot laboratory is

    a. hourly.   c. weekly.
    b. daily.   d. monthly.

25. Misadministration of radioactive material includes which of the following?

    1. improper quantity of radioactive material
    2. improper radioisotope
    3. improper route of administration
    4. excessive dose

    a. Only 1, 2, and 3 are correct.
    b. Only 1 and 3 are correct.
    c. Only 2 and 4 are correct.
    d. All are correct.

26. Effective radioactive waste disposal includes segregation of such waste by

    a. form (liquid-solid).
    b. emission energy.
    c. half-life.
    d. volatility.

27. Which of the following instruments is most helpful for contamination control?
    a. thermoluminescent dosimeter
    b. Geiger counter
    c. ionization chamber
    d. film badge

28. The recommended frequency of wipe tests in an imaging laboratory is
    a. hourly.   c. weekly.
    b. daily.   d. monthly.

29. Following a study involving ^{99m}Tc, a nursing mother should discontinue breast feeding for
    a. 1 day   c. 1 week
    b. 2 days   d. 1 month

30. Which of the following is considered short-lived radioactive waste?
    a. ^{99m}Tc   c. ^{131}I
    b. ^{67}Ga   d. ^{111}In

Chapter 9 Practice Questions (Diagnostic Ultrasound Imaging)

1. The two general types of responses to ultrasound exposure are
   a. ionization-excitation.
   b. cavitation-excitation.
   c. ionization-polarization.
   d. thermal-nonthermal.

2. Which of the following is the most important factor affecting the thermal response to diagnostic ultrasound?
   a. temporal average intensity
   b. temporal peak intensity
   c. pulse repetition frequency
   d. length of exposure

3. Ultrasound absorption increases with
   a. increasing frequency.
   b. increasing wavelength.
   c. reduced focal length.
   d. reduced pulse length.

4. An ultrasonographer can perform an examination ALARA by
   1. maintaining a low output intensity.
   2. selecting the lowest appropriate frequency.
   3. selecting the lowest appropriate pulse repetition frequency.
   4. selecting the longest appropriate pulse length.

    a. Only 1, 2, and 3 are correct.

    b. Only 1 and 3 are correct.

    c. Only 2 and 4 are correct.

    d. All are correct.

5. The scanning indexes available on an ultrasound imager console have a scale of

    a. 0 to 5.   c. 1 to 4.

    b. 0 to 10.   d. 1 to 8.

6. Which of the following is a nonthermal tissue response to ultrasound?

    a. temperature rise   c. excitation

    b. cavitation   d. polarization

7. Which of the following contributes to ultrasound attenuation?

    a. excitation   c. polarization

    b. ionization   d. absorption

8. Ultrasound that penetrates deeper into tissue is that with a

    a. higher frequency.

    b. longer wavelength.

    c. longer pulse length.

    d. higher pulse repetition frequency.

9. Which of the following is an example of ALARA in diagnostic ultrasound?

    a. increasing time gain control rather than beam intensity

    b. selecting the highest frequency transducer appropriate to the examination

    c. selecting the longest pulse length appropriate to the examination

    d. using the highest pulse repetition frequency appropriate to the examination

10. Which of the following should be implemented when nuclear medicine patients are referred to diagnostic ultrasound?

    1. providing the ultrasonographer with a film badge

    2. using disposable gowns, pads, and utensils

    3. performing a contamination survey after the examination

    4. taking no special precautions

    a. Only 1, 2, and 3 are correct.

    b. Only 1 and 3 are correct.

    c. Only 2 and 4 are correct.

    d. Only 4 is correct.

11. Which of the following is a mechanical response to ultrasound exposure?

    a. membrane shearing

    b. excitation

    c. thermal induction

    d. electric conduction

12. Which of the following contributes to ultrasound attenuation?

    a. beam scattering   c. beam steering

    b. beam focusing   d. beam sweeping

13. The principal tissue of concern in diagnostic ultrasound imaging is
    a. waterlike, such as cerebrospinal fluid.
    b. cartilage.
    c. adult bone.
    d. fetal bone.

14. Which of the following is designed to warn of nonthermal effects?
    a. mechanical index (MI)
    b. soft tissue thermal index (TIS)
    c. cranial bone thermal index (TIC)
    d. bone thermal index (TIB)

15. Ultrasound intensity is measured in
    a. milliwatts (mW).
    b. milliwatts per centimeter squared (mW/cm²)
    c. milliwatts per second (mW/s).
    d. watts per second (W/s).

16. The ultrasound absorption coefficient has units of
    a. dB.   c. dB/cm/MHz.
    b. dB/cm.   d. dB/cm/MHz/s

17. Which of the following diagrams represents heating of homogeneous soft tissue such as abdomen?
    a. A   c. C
    b. B   d. D

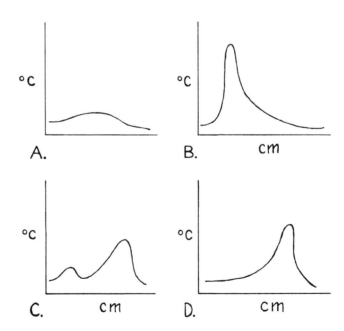

18. Which of the following is designed to guard against temperature increases in muscle?
    a. mechanical index (MI)
    b. soft tissue thermal index (TIS)
    c. cranial bone thermal index (TIC)
    d. bone thermal index (TIB)

19. The thermal effects of ultrasound beams occur most readily
    a. at the transducer skin interface.
    b. on the skin.
    c. just beneath the skin.
    d. at the depth of focus.

20. Which of the following tissues has the lowest absorption coefficient?
    a. fetal bone   c. water
    b. adult bone   d. muscle

21. Which of the following represents heating of soft tissue distal to a fluid-filled bladder?
    a. A   c. C
    b. B   d. D

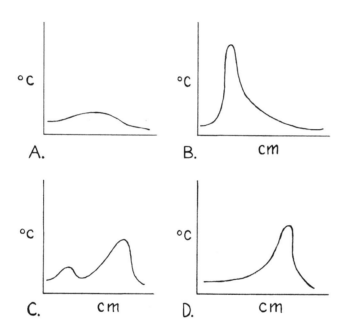

22. Which of the following is designed to guard against unnecessary fetal bone exposure?
    a. mechanical index (MI)
    b. soft tissue thermal index (TIS)
    c. cranial bone thermal index (TIC)
    d. bone thermal index (TIB)

23. The thermal effects of diagnostic ultrasound are principally a function of
    a. pulse length.
    b. pulse repetition frequency.
    c. temporal average intensity.
    d. temporal peak intensity.

24. Which of the following tissues has the highest absorption coefficient?
    a. fetal bone   c. water
    b. skin   d. cartilage

25. Which of the following represents the heating of fetal bone at a depth?

    a. A   c. C
    b. B   d. D

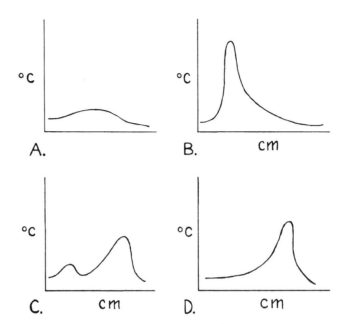

26. Which of the following best indicates the potential for heating of bone near the surface?

    a. mechanical index (MI)
    b. soft tissue thermal index (TIS)
    c. cranial bone thermal index (TIC)
    d. bone thermal index (TIB)

27. Which of the following tissues is likely to experience the greatest temperature rise following ultrasound exposure?

    a. water   c. muscle
    b. fetal bone   d. skin

28. The principal nonthermal response to diagnostic ultrasound is

    a. ionization.   c. polarization.
    b. excitation.   d. cavitation.

Chapter 9 Practice Questions (Magnetic Resonance Imaging)

1. Which electromagnetic radiation is used for magnetic resonance imaging?

    a. γ rays
    b. microwaves
    c. radio frequencies
    d. magnetic waves

2. The range of the electromagnetic spectrum employed for MRI is approximately

    a. 1 to 10 MHz.   c. 300 to 500 nm.
    b. 10 to 100 MHz.   d. 500 to 800 nm.

3. Which of the following are transient magnetic fields?

   1. B_0
   2. RF
   3. RF/s
   4. B_z

   a. Only 1, 2, and 3 are correct.
   b. Only 1 and 3 are correct.
   c. Only 2 and 4 are correct.
   d. Only 4 is correct.

4. The principal interaction between the B_0 field and soft tissue is

   a. ionization.
   b. excitation.
   c. polarization.
   d. thermalization.

5. Which of the following represents a response of the heart to magnetic resonance imaging?

   a. magnetophosphenes
   b. peripheral stimulation
   c. ventricular fibrillation
   d. cardiac arrest

6. When averaged over the anatomy of interest, the maximum SAR permitted for clinical MRI in the United States is

   a. 1 W/kg.
   b. 2 W/kg.
   c. 4 W/kg.
   d. 8 W/kg.

7. The principal hazard to the public from MRI is due to

   a. the B_0 field.
   b. the B_{xyz} fields.
   c. RF emission.
   d. projectiles.

8. MRI should not be conducted on which of the following?

   a. a patient with a prosthetic hip
   b. a pregnant patient
   c. a newborn
   d. a patient with a cardiac pacemaker

9. The radiation used to create magnetic resonance images is positioned where along the electromagnetic spectrum?

   a. at a long wavelength
   b. at a heavy mass
   c. at a slow velocity
   d. at high energy

10. The range of the electromagnetic spectrum employed for MRI is approximately

    1. 1 to 10 keV.
    2. 10 to 100 keV.
    3. 1 to 10 MHz.
    4. 10 to 100 MHz.

    a. Only 1, 2, and 3 are correct.
    b. Only 1 and 3 are correct.
    c. Only 2 and 4 are correct.
    d. Only 4 is correct.

11. Which of the following MRI fields interacts with tissue thermally?

    a. RF
    b. B_0
    c. B_{xyz}
    d. B_z

12. When a patient is exposed to the B_0 field,
    a. nothing happens, even at the molecular level.
    b. polarization occurs, but only during such exposure.
    c. polarization can last for several hours after exposure.
    d. polarization is permanent.

13. Which of the following represents the principal hazard encountered during routine MRI?
    a. projectiles   c. cataracts
    b. magnetophosphenes d. superficial burns

14. The maximum SAR permitted for clinical MRI is the value that should limit tissue heating to approximately
    a. 0.5°C.   c. 3°C.
    b. 1°C.   d. 5°C.

15. Those members of the public requiring the most protection during MRI are those
    a. with surgical clips.
    b. with implanted prostheses.
    c. with cardiac pacemakers.
    d. who are wheelchair-bound.

16. A pregnant MRI technologist should
    a. be reassigned to a non-MRI job.
    b. not be allowed in the imaging room.
    c. not be allowed to stand immediately next to the magnet for an extended time.
    d. continue her normal work assignments.

17. The radiation used to create magnetic resonance images is positioned where along the electromagnetic spectrum?
    a. at a short wavelength
    b. at a low frequency
    c. at a slow velocity
    d. at high energy

18. The intensity of RF radiation is measured in
    a. tesla (T).
    b. megahertz (MHz).
    c. watts (W).
    d. watts per kilogram (W/kg).

19. Which of the following MR imaging fields can raise the temperature of tissue?
    1. B_0 3. B_z
    2. B_{xyz} 4. RF
    a. Only 1, 2, and 3 are correct.
    b. Only 1 and 3 are correct.
    c. Only 2 and 4 are correct.
    d. Only 4 is correct.

20. The principal interaction between transient magnetic fields and soft tissue is
    a. ionization.
    b. polarization.
    c. electrical induction.
    d. thermal induction.

21. If a surgical clip twists during MRI, the energy field causing such twisting is most likely
    a. RF.
    b. B_{xy}.
    c. B_z.
    d. B_0.

22. A limitation is placed on the SAR in clinical MRI because of concerns about
    a. ionization.
    b. excitation.
    c. peripheral nerve stimulation.
    d. tissue heating.

23. The intensity-response relationship for the RF field employed in MRI is best described as
    1. hazardous.
    2. totally safe.
    3. nonthreshold.
    4. threshold.
    a. Only 1, 2, and 3 are correct.
    b. Only 1 and 3 are correct.
    c. Only 2 and 4 are correct.
    d. Only 4 is correct.

24. The radiation used to create magnetic resonance images is positioned where along the electromagnetic spectrum?
    a. at a short wavelength
    b. at a high frequency
    c. at high velocity
    d. at low energy

25. The intensity of the B_0 field is measured in
    a. tesla (T).
    b. megahertz (MHz).
    c. watts (W).
    d. watts per kilogram (W/kg).

26. What minimal RF intensity is required to raise the temperature of soft tissue approximately 1°C?
    a. 0.1 to 0.5 W/kg
    b. 1 to 5 W/kg
    c. 10 to 50 W/kg
    d. 100 to 500 W/kg

27. The following have been reported as responses to gradient magnetic field exposure
    1. sensory nerve stimulation
    2. bone heating
    3. peripheral nerve stimulation
    4. soft tissue heating
    a. Only 1, 2, and 3 are correct.
    b. Only 1 and 3 are correct.
    c. Only 2 and 4 are correct.
    d. All are correct.

28. Projectiles in an MRI room can be created by which of the following fields?

a. B_0

b. B_{xyz}

c. RF

d. B_z

29. Exposure of pregnant MRI operators to the B_0 field is

a. limited to 0.5 T.

b. limited to 1 T.

c. limited to 2 T.

d. unlimited.

30. The intensity-response relationship for the B_0 field employed in MRI is best described as

1. hazardous.

2. totally safe.

3. nonthreshold.

4. threshold.

a. Only 1, 2, and 3 are correct.

b. Only 1 and 3 are correct.

c. Only 2 and 4 are correct.

d. Only 4 is correct.

31. The radiation used to create magnetic resonance images is positioned where along the eletromagnetic spectrum?

1. at a short wavelength

2. at a low frequency

3. at high velocity

4. at low energy

a. Only 1, 2 and 3 are correct.

b. Only 1 and 3 are correct.

c. Only 2 and 4 are correct.

d. All are correct.

32. Which of the following magnetic resonance energy fields remains constant in intensity during imaging?

a. B_0

b. B_{xy}

c. B_z

d. RF

33. Regarding RF heating of soft tissue,

1. the more vascular the tissue, the less the temperature rise.

2. the deeper the tissue, the greater the temperature rise.

3. the longer the exposure, the greater the temperature rise.

4. the higher the temperature, the more likely is ionization.

a. Only 1, 2, and 3 are correct.

b. Only 1 and 3 are correct.

c. Only 2 and 4 are correct.

d. All are correct.

34. Which of the following can occur as a result of exposure to Bxy?

a. neuronal conduction

b. tissue heating

c. cataract formation

d. ionization

35. In the United States, which federal agency is responsible for MRI safety?

    a. Department of Energy
    b. Food and Drug Administration
    c. Nuclear Regulatory Commission
    d. National Institutes of Health

36. Exposure of pregnant operators to the transient magnetic fields during MRI is

    a. limited to 10 T/s.   c. limited to 40 T/s.
    b. limited to 20 T/s.   d. unlimited.

37. The intensity-response relationship for the B_{xyz} fields employed in MRI is best described as

    1. hazardous.   3. nonthreshold.
    2. totally safe.   4. threshold.

    a. Only 1, 2 and 3 are correct.
    b. Only 1 and 3 are correct.
    c. Only 2 and 4 are correct.
    d. Only 4 is correct.

38. The range of the electromagnetic spectrum employed for MRI is approximately

    a. 1 to 10 MHz.   c. 100 to 500 MHz.
    b. 10 to 100 MHz.   d. 500 to 1,000 MHz.

39. Which of the following energy fields are measured in T/s?

    1. B_0 3. RF
    2. B_{xy} 4. B_z
    a. Only 1, 2, and 3 are correct.
    b. Only 1 and 3 are correct.
    c. Only 2 and 4 are correct.
    d. Only 4 is correct.

40. Which of the following can result from irradiation of the head with RF?

    a. bone cancer   c. erythema
    b. leukemia   d. cataracts

41. Which of the following are suspected patient responses to transient magnetic fields?

    1. magnetophosphenes 3. metallic taste
    2. twitching   4. ventricular fibrillation

    a. Only 1, 2, and 3 are correct.
    b. Only 1 and 3 are correct.
    c. Only 2 and 4 are correct.
    d. All are correct.

42. In the United States, the maximum intensity B_0 permitted for clinical imaging is

    a. 0.1 T.   c. 2 T.
    b. 1 T.   d. 4 T.

43. Exposure of pregnant MRI operators to the radio-frequency field is
    a. limited to 1 W/kg.
    b. limited to 2 W/kg.
    c. limited to 4 W/kg.
    d. unlimited.

44. Approximately what percentage of patients have been reported claustrophobic and unable to be imaged with MRI?
    a. 1   c. 10
    b. 5   d. 20

45. Which of the following is a transient magnetic field?
    a. B_0 c. RF
    b. B_z d. RF/s

46. Which of the following best describes light flashes that appear while the eyes are closed?
    a. magnetocisterns
    b. magnetophosphenes
    c. RF stimulation
    d. RF thermalization

47. In the United States, the maximum intensity permitted for transient magnetic fields is
    a. 2 T/s.   c. 40 T/s.
    b. 20 T/s.   d. 60 T/s.

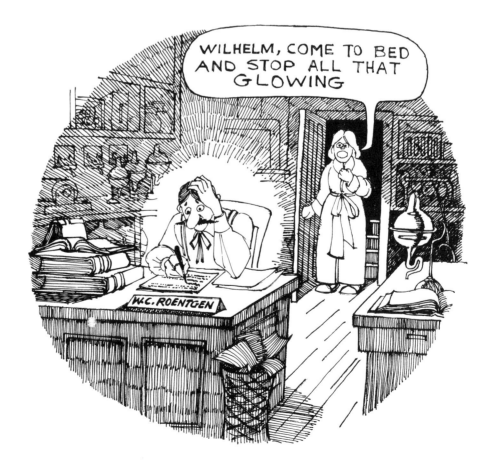

Appendices

Glossary

A mode (amplitude mode) Method of ultrasound signal display in which time is represented along the horizontal axis and echo amplitude is displayed along the vertical axis.

Absolute risk Incidence of malignant disease in a population within 1 year for a given dose. Expressed as number of cases/106 persons/rem.

Absorbed dose **a.** Energy transferred from ionizing radiation per unit mass of irradiated material. Expressed in rad (100 erg/g) or gray (1 J/kg). **b.** Thermalization of tissue by absorption of ultrasound energy. Expressed as temperature rise (°C).

Absorber Any material that absorbs or reduces the intensity of radiation.

Absorption **a.** Transfer of energy from an electromagnetic field to matter. Removal of x rays from a beam via the photoelectric effect. **b.** Process by which ultrasound transfers energy to tissue by conversion of acoustic energy to heat.

Accommodation Ability of the eye to change its power and thus focus for different object distances.

Acids Hydrogen-containing compounds that can attack and dissolve metal.

Acoustic attenuation Reduction of ultrasound beam intensity by absorption, scattering, reflection, refraction, or diffraction.

Acoustic energy Mechanical energy transported by an ultrasound beam. Expressed as the product of acoustic power and time (Ws). 1 Ws = 1 J.

Acoustic impedance **a.** Ratio of instantaneous ultrasound pressure at a tissue interface to its velocity at that interface. **b.** Product of ultrasound velocity v in a tissue of mass density r. Expressed in rayls where 1 rayl = $(kg/m^2 \; s)(10^{-6})$.

Acoustic impedance match Condition of nearly equal acoustic impedance of contiguous media in order to avoid reflection of acoustic energy at the interface.

Acoustic intensity Ultrasonic power transmitted per unit area. Expressed in mW/cm^2.

Acoustic lens Refractive element employed to redirect an ultrasound beam in order to increase or decrease ultrasound intensity or to focus the beam.

Acoustic power Acoustic energy per unit time. Expressed in W or J/s.

Acoustic pressure Instantaneous value of total pressure minus ambient pressure.

Acoustic shadow Manifestation of reduced ultrasound intensity in or returning from regions lying beyond an attenuating object. Different than in regions of low reflectivity.

Acoustic streaming Acoustically generated transport of fluid within sonified tissue.

Acoustic wave Mechanical disturbance that propagates through a medium.

Acoustic wavelength **a.** Distance between any two similar adjacent points of an ultrasound wave. **b.** Distance traveled by a sound wave during one cycle.

Acoustics **a.** Science of sound, including its production, transmission, and effects. **b.** Containing, producing, arising from, actuated by, related to, or associated with sound or ultrasound.

Activity (See Radioactivity).

Acute Beginning suddenly and running a short but rather severe course.

Acute effects (See Early effects).

Acute radiation syndrome Radiation sickness that occurs in humans after whole-body doses of 1 Gy (100 rad) or more of ionizing radiation delivered over a short period of time.

Added filtration Aluminum (or its equivalent) of appropriate thickness positioned outside the glass window of an x-ray tube and in the primary beam.

Agreement states Individual states that have entered into agreement with the United States Nuclear Regulatory Commission (USNRC) to enforce radiation protection regulations dealing with radioactive material.

ALARA The principle that radiation exposure should be kept as low as reasonably achievable, economic and social factors being taken into account.

Algorithm Computer-adapted mathematical calculation applied to raw data during the process of image reconstruction.

Alpha particle (α particle)
Particulate form of ionizing radiation consisting of two protons and two neutrons. The nucleus of helium. Emitted from the nucleus of a radioactive atom.

Alternating current Oscillation of electrons in both directions in a conductor.

Aluminum (Al) Metal most frequently selected as x-ray beam filter material because it effectively removes low-energy x rays.

Aluminum equivalent Thickness of a material resulting in the same attenuation as aluminum.

American Association of Physicists in Medicine (AAPM) Scientific society of medical physicists.

American College of Medical Physicists (ACMP) Professional society of medical physicists.

American College of Radiology (ACR) Professional society of radiologists and medical physicists.

American Society of Radiologic Technologists (ASRT) Scientific and professional society of radiographers.

Amino acids Structural units of protein.

Ampere (A) The SI unit of electric charge. 1 A = 1 C/s.

Amplitude Magnitude of the waveform of an acoustic, electric, or electromagnetic signal.

Analog signal Continuous display of energy, intensity, or radiation, as opposed to the discrete display of a digital signal.

Anaphase Second phase of mitosis during which chromatids repel each other and migrate along the mitotic spindle to opposite sides of the cell.

Anemia Condition characterized by a lack of vitality and caused by a decrease in the number of red blood cells.

Angle of incidence Angle between the axis of an ultrasound beam at an interface and the perpendicular to the interface.

Angstrom (Å) Unit of measure of wavelength. 1 Å = 10^{-10} m.

Anion Negatively charged ion.

Anisotropic Having different intensities in different directions.

Annihilation radiation Two 0.511-keV γ rays emitted in opposite directions, resulting from the interaction of a positron and an electron.

Annotation Text added to images to provide descriptions or labeling.

Anode Positively charged side of an x-ray tube which contains the target.

Antenna Device for transmitting or receiving electromagnetic radiation.

Antibodies Proteins produced by the body in response to the presence of foreign antigens such as bacteria or viruses.

Aperture a. Circular opening for the patient in the gantry of a CT or magnetic resonance imager. b. Fixed collimation of a diagnostic x-ray tube as in an aperture diaphragm. c. Variable opening before the lens of a cine- or photospot camera.

Aplastic anemia Anemia resulting from bone marrow failure.

Archival storage Secondary or permanent storage of digital images—usually magnetic tapes, magnetic disks, or optical disks—and film images.

Array processor Part of a computer that handles raw data and performs the mathematical calculations necessary to reconstruct a digital image.

Artifacts Patterns on an image that do not represent anatomy.

Atom Smallest particle of an element that cannot be divided or broken up by chemical means.

Atomic mass number (A) Number of protons plus number of neutrons in the nucleus.

Atomic number (Z) Number of protons in the nucleus.

Attenuation Reduction in radiation intensity when passing through matter as a result of absorption and scattering (See Acoustic attenuation).

Attenuation coefficient Numerical expression of the decrease in intensity with distance or penetration. The x-ray attenuation coefficient is expressed in inverse length (m^{-1}, cm^{-1}). The ultrasound attenuation coefficient is expressed in dB/cm.

Attenuator Device that reduces x-ray or ultrasound intensity.

Axial resolution Minimum separation of reflectors along an ultrasound beam that can be separately distinguished.

Axon Extension fiber from a nerve cell body that conducts impulses.

Azimuthal resolution (See Lateral resolution).

B mode Method of ultrasound image display in which the intensity of the echo is represented by brightness and its location displayed in the xy plane is determined by the position of the transducer.

Background radiation Radiation exposure from cosmic sources. Naturally occurring radioactive materials and radioactive material internally deposited in the body.

Backscatter X rays that have interacted with an object and are deflected in a backward direction.

Bandwidth Range of frequencies contained in a RF or ultrasound pulse.

Base Alkali or alkaline earth OH compounds that can neutralize acids.

Beam axis Central line representing maximum ultrasound or x-ray intensity.

Beam limiting device Device that provides a means to restrict the size of an x-ray field (See Collimator).

Beam width Transverse distance of useful ultrasound or x-ray intensity on a specified beam cross-sectional profile.

Becquerel (Bq) Special name for the SI unit of radioactivity. 1 Bq = 1 disintegration/s.

Beta particle (β particle) Ionizing radiation with characteristics of an electron. Emitted from the nucleus of a radioactive atom.

Binding energy Energy that holds the nucleus of an atom together and the electrons to the nucleus.

Black body Ideal body that is in thermal equilibrium with the electromagnetic energy incident on it. It behaves as if the incident energy is completely absorbed.

Bone seeker A radioisotope that tends to accumulate in the bones when injected (e.g., ^{90}Sr and ^{226}Ra).

Brachytherapy Radiation oncology in which the source of radiation is on or in the body.

Bremsstrahlung X-rays produced by deceleration of electrons near the nucleus of a target atom.

Brightness mode (See B mode).

C-arm fluoroscope Portable device for fluoroscopy. The opposite ends of the "C" support arm hold the image intensifier and the x-ray tube.

Calibration Comparison of a laboratory source or instrument in daily use with a standard source or instrument to improve accuracy.

Carbohydrates Compounds composed entirely of carbon, hydrogen, and oxygen.

Carbon Nonmetallic element that is the basic constituent of all organic matter.

Carcinogenic Causing cancer.

Catalyst Molecule that affects the speed of a chemical reaction without being altered itself.

Cataractogenic Causing cataracts.

Cataracts Clouding of the lens that obstructs vision.

Cathode Negatively charged source of electrons in an x-ray tube.

Cathode ray tube (CRT) Electron beam tube designed for a two-dimensional display of signals. A TV picture tube.

Cation Positively charged ion.

Cavitation Phenomenon caused by high-intensity ultrasound in tissue, resulting in bubbles or cavities containing gas or vapor.

Cell Basic unit of all living matter.

Cell division Process whereby one cell divides to form two or more cells.

Cell membrane Structure encasing and surrounding a cell.

Cell metabolism Biochemical reactions necessary for cellular function, growth, and reproduction.

Center for Devices and Radiological Health (CDRH) Known as the Bureau of Radiological Health (BRH) before 1982. Responsible for a national electronic radiation control program.

Center frequency Middle frequency of the frequency bandwidth. Generally, the frequency at which the RF or ultrasound amplitude is a maximum.

Centigray 0.01 Gy.

Central nervous system syndrome Form of acute radiation syndrome caused by radiation doses of 50 Gy (5,000 rad) or more of ionizing radiation that results in failure of the central nervous system followed by death within a few hours to several days.

Centromere Clear region on a chromosome where its arms join.

Characteristic x rays X rays released as a result of the photoelectric effect whose discrete energies are determined by the respective electron binding energy.

Charged particle An ion. Elementary particle carrying a positive or negative electric charge.

Chromatid One of the two duplicate portions of DNA that appears as an arm of a chromosome.

Chromosomal aberrations Visible changes in chromosome structure.

Chromosomes Small, rod-shaped bodies containing genes.

Chronic Continuing for a long time, as in disease or radiation exposure.

Cinefluorography Recording of fluoroscopic images on movie film.

Classical scattering Scattering of x rays with no loss of energy. Also called **coherent**, **Rayleigh**, or **Thompson scattering**.

Coefficient of variation Standard deviation divided by the value measured.

Coherent scattering (See Classical scattering).

Collimation Restriction of the useful x-ray beam to the anatomical area of interest.

Collimator Device to restrict the size and shape of an x-ray beam.

Compensating filter Material inserted between an x-ray source and a patient to shape the intensity of the x-ray beam. X-ray beam filter designed to make the remnant beam more uniform in intensity.

Compound Chemical combination of two or more elements in fixed and definite proportions.

Compton electron Electron emitted from the outer shell of an atom as a result of x-ray interaction.

Compton scattering Interaction between an x ray and a loosely bound outer-shell electron, resulting in ionization and x-ray scattering.

Computed tomography (CT) Creation of a cross-sectional tomographic section of the body using a rotating fan beam, detector array, and computed reconstruction.

Conductor Material that allows heat or electric current to flow relatively easily.

Cone Circular metal tube that attaches to x-ray tube housing to limit the beam size and shape.

Congenital abnormalities Defects existing at birth that were not inherited but rather were acquired during development in utero.

Contact coupling Acoustic coupling using gel or liquid to exclude air from the space between the transducer and the skin.

Continuous wave (CW) Ultrasound wave of constant amplitude which persists for a large number of cycles.

Contrast resolution Ability to detect and display similar tissues such as gray matter and white matter and liver and spleen.

Control badge Personnel radiation monitor provided with each batch of badges to allow determination of exposure while in transit.

Control chart Graphical plot of quality control test results with respect to time or sequence of measurement along with acceptance limits.

Control limits Limits shown on a control chart beyond which performance is compromised and corrective action required.

Controlled area Area where personnel occupancy and activity are subject to control and supervision for the purpose of radiation protection. Such personnel usually wear personnel radiation monitors.

Cosmic radiation Penetrating ionizing radiation, both particulate and electromagnetic, originating in outer space.

Coulomb (C) SI unit of electric charge.

Coulomb per kilogram (C/kg) SI unit of radiation exposure. 2.58×10^{-4} C/kg = 1 R.

Covalent bond Chemical union between atoms formed by sharing one or more pairs of electrons.

Critical organ Body organ receiving a radiation dose or radionuclide that results in the greatest overall damage to the body.

Crossover Process occurring during meiosis when chromatids exchange chromosomal material.

Crystal Colloquial term for the piezoelectric element of an ultrasound transducer.

Cumulative timing device Device that measures the on time of a fluoroscopic x-ray beam and alarms at 5 min.

Curie (Ci) Former unit of radioactivity. Expressed as 1 Ci = 3.7×10^{10} disintegrations/s = 3.7×10^{10} Bq.

Cursor Electronic pointer used to outline areas of interest on a digital image for analysis. Used to highlight all the pixels of an area.

Cutie pie Nickname for an ionization chamber-type survey meter.

Cytoplasm Protoplasm existing outside the cell's nucleus.

Damping Any material or mechanism that removes mechanical motion from an ultrasound transducer. Used to improve axial resolution.

Dead-man-type fluoroscopic exposure switch Exposure switch (operated by foot pressure) that requires continuous pressure applied by the operator. Should the operator die, exposure will cease—unless the operator falls on the switch!

Dead time Time interval between the beginning of an ultrasound pulse and the arrival of the first echo.

Decibel (dB) a. Ten times the logarithm to the base 10 of the ratio of two intensities. b. One-tenth of a bel. c. Used to express the ratio of two like quantities such as RF signals or transmitted and reflected ultrasound.

Declared pregnancy Referred to in a voluntary statement made by a woman informing her employer, in writing, of her pregnancy and the estimated date of conception.

Deep-dose equivalent (H_d) Applies to external whole-body exposure. The dose equivalent at a tissue depth of 1 cm.

Densitometer Instrument that measures the optical density of exposed film.

Deoxyribonucleic acid (DNA) Molecule that carries the genetic information necessary for cell replication. The target molecule of radiobiology.

Depth of focus Distance along an ultrasound beam axis where the beam cross-sectional area is minimum.

Detector Device or material that is sensitive to x rays.

Detector array Group of detectors and the interspace material used to separate them. The image receptor in computed tomography.

Deterministic effects Biological responses whose severity varies with radiation dose. A dose threshold usually exists.

Diagnostic-type protective tube housing Lead-lined housing enclosing an x-ray tube that shields leakage radiation to less than 100 mR/h at 1 m.

Diaphragm Device that restricts an x-ray beam to a fixed size.

Dicentric chromosomes Chromosomes having two centromeres.

Diffuse reflection Occurs when an ultrasound beam incident on a surface is reflected over a wide range of angles, as opposed to specular reflection.

Diffusion Motion of gas, liquid, or solid particles from an area of relatively high concentration to an area of lower concentration.

Dipole antenna RF antenna that produces or receives a signal approximating an elementary electric dipole. An antenna constructed of a single length of conductor.

Direct current Flow of electrons in only one direction in a conductor.

Direct effect Effect of ionizing radiation interacting directly with the target molecule, DNA.

Disintegration (See Radioactive decay).

Display format Matter in which the ultrasound image is presented (A mode, B mode, C mode, etc.).

Dominant mutation Genetic mutation that will probably be expressed in offspring.

Doppler effect Shift in observed frequency caused by relative motions among sources and/or receivers.

Doppler shift frequency Difference between the frequencies of transmitted and received ultrasound.

Doppler ultrasound Application of the Doppler effect in ultrasound to detect wall movement, as in cardiac imaging, or blood flow, as in vascular imaging.

Dose Amount of energy absorbed by an irradiated object per unit mass.

Dose equivalent (*H*) Radiation quantity used for radiation protection purposes that expresses dose on a common scale for all radiations. Expressed in rem or sievert (Sv).

Dosimeter Instrument for detecting and measuring exposure to ionizing radiation.

Dosimetry Theory and application of principles and techniques involved in the measurement and recording of radiation dose. Quantitative determination of spatial and temporal radiation exposure.

Doubling dose Dose of radiation expected to double the number of spontaneous mutations in a generation.

Duty cycle Ratio of on time to total exposure duration of pulsed ultrasound imaging.

Duty factor Product of ultrasound pulse duration and pulse repetition rate.

Dynamic imaging Imaging of an object in motion. Imaging in real time (See Fluoroscopy).

Early effects Effects of ionizing radiation that appear within weeks of the time of exposure. Also called **acute effects**.

Echo Ultrasound received from the specular reflection at a tissue interface.

Effective atomic number Weighted average atomic number for the different elements of a material.

Effective dose (*E*) Sum over specified tissues of the products of the equivalent dose in a tissue (H_T) and the weighting factor for that tissue (W_T) (i.e., $E = \Sigma W_T H_T$).

Effective dose equivalent (H_E) Sum of the products of the dose equivalent to a tissue (H_T) and the weighting factors (W_T) applicable to each of the tissues irradiated (i.e., $H_E = \Sigma W_T H_T$). The values of W_T are different for effective dose and effective dose equivalent.

Electric dipole Pair of equal and opposite charges separated by an infinitesimal distance. When the charges are oscillating, the dipole becomes an elementary radiating electric dipole.

Electric potential energy Electrical energy acquired by a charged particle as a result of its position relative to other charged particles. Expressed in joules (J).

Electromagnetic radiation X-rays, γ rays, and some nonionizing radiation such as ultraviolet, visible, infrared, and radio waves. Oscillating electric and magnetic fields that travel in a vacuum with the velocity of light.

Electromagnetic spectrum Continuum of electromagnetic radiation.

Electrometer Device used to measure electric charge.

Electromotive force Electric potential. Expressed in volts (V).

Electron Elementary particle with one negative charge. Electrons surround the positively charged nucleus and determine the chemical properties of the atom.

Electron volt (eV) Unit of energy equal to that which an electron acquires from a potential difference of 1 V.

Element Atoms having the same atomic number and same chemical properties. A substance that cannot be broken down further without changing its chemical properties.

Emaciation State of being extremely thin.

Embryo Developing human from conception through approximately 8 weeks.

Embryo or fetus Developing human from conception until birth.

Embryological effects Damage occurring as a result of an organism being exposed to ionizing radiation during its embryonic stage of development.

Endoplasmic reticulum Vast, irregular network of tubules and vesicles spreading in all directions throughout the cytoplasm.

Energy Ability to do work. Expressed in joules (J).

Entrance skin exposure (ESE) X-ray exposure of the skin. Expressed in mR.

Envelope Continuous curve connecting the peaks of the successive cycles of a waveform, as in a free induction decay or spin echo.

Epilation Loss of hair.

Epithelial tissue Tissue that covers the body and organs. It is highly radiosensitive.

Equivalent dose (See Dose equivalent).

Erg Unit of energy and work.

Error Difference between the measured value and the true value of a parameter or quantity.

Erythroblasts Red blood stem cells.

Erythrocytes Red blood cells.

Excitation Addition of energy to a system. Raising the energy of electrons with the use of x rays.

Exposure Measure of the ionization produced in air by x or γ rays. Amount of ionizing radiation to which an object such as a human body may be subjected. Quantity of radiation intensity. Expressed in R, C/kg, or air kerma Gy.

Exposure linearity Consistency in radiation intensity stated in mR/mAs when changing from one mA station to the next.

Exposure reproducibility Consistency in radiation intensity from an individual exposure to subsequent exposures with the same technique.

Exposure time a. Total time an ultrasound transducer delivers ultrasonic energy to a patient. In a pulse waveform this includes time between pulses. b. The time an x-ray tube is energized and a useful beam produced.

Extremity Hand, elbow, or arm below the elbow, and foot, knee, or leg below the knee.

Eye dose equivalent External exposure of the lens of the eye. Taken as the dose equivalent at a tissue depth of 0.3 cm (300 mg/cm^3).

Far field The region of an ultrasound beam in which the acoustic energy along the beam axis diverges as though coming from a point source located near the transducer assembly.

Fast fission Fission of a heavy atom such as ^{238}U when it absorbs a high-energy (fast) neutron. Most fissionable materials require thermal (slow) neutrons.

Fats Compounds composed of carbon, hydrogen, and oxygen with the hydrogen/oxygen ratio being very much greater than 2:1.

Fetus Developing human from approximately the ninth week of pregnancy until birth.

Filament That part of the cathode that emits electrons resulting in x-ray tube current.

Film badge Most widely used and most economical type of personnel radiation monitor. Pack of photographic film used for approximate measurement of radiation exposure to radiation workers.

Filter Added material that increases x-ray effective energy by absorbing low-energy x rays. Device designed to reduce patient dose.

Filtration Removal of low-energy x rays from the useful beam with aluminum or other metal. Results in increased beam quality and reduced patient dose.

Fission Splitting of a nucleus into at least two other nuclei and release of a relatively large amount of energy and two or three neutrons.

Fluoroscopy X-ray imaging in real time.

Focal length Axial distance from a focusing ultrasound transducer to the depth of minimum beam area.

Focal spot Area of the anode where x rays are actually produced.

Focal zone Volume of tissue including the depth of focus where there is the best lateral ultrasound resolution.

Focusing transducer assembly Ultrasound transducer assembly which can be electronically focused at multiple depths in tissue.

Force That which changes the motion of an object. A push or pull. Expressed in newtons (N).

Fraunhofer zone (See Far field).

Free radicals Very reactive chemical molecules with unpaired electrons in the valence or outermost shell.

Frequency Number of cycles or wavelengths of a simple harmonic motion per unit time. Expressed in Hertz (Hz). 1 Hz = 1 cycle/s.

Fresnel zone (See Near field).

Fusion A thermonuclear reaction characterized by joining together of light nuclei to form heavier nuclei.

Gadolinium Rare-earth element used in intensifying screens and MRI contrast agents.

Gain Ratio of output to input of an amplifying system. Expressed in decibels (dB).

Gamma ray (γ ray) High-energy, short-wavelength electromagnetic radiation emitted from the nucleus during radioactive decay.

Gantry Portion of the CT or magnetic resonance imager that accommodates the patient and source or detector assemblies.

Gastrointestinal (GI) syndrome Form of acute radiation syndrome that appears in humans at a threshold dose of about 10 Gy (1,000 rad).

Geiger-Müeller (G-M) counter Radiation detection and measuring instrument that detects individual ionizations. The primary radiation survey instrument for nuclear medicine facilities.

Genes Basic units of heredity.

Genetic effect Effect in a descendant resulting from the modification of genetic material in a parent. Radiation damage to generations yet unborn.

Genetically significant dose (GSD) Average annual gonadal dose to members of the population who are of childbearing age.

Germ cells Reproductive cells.

Gonadal shield Device used during radiologic procedures to protect the reproductive organs from exposure to the useful beam when they are in or within about 5 cm of a collimated beam.

Gray (Gy) Special name for the SI unit of absorbed dose and air kerma. 1 Gy = 1 J/kg = 100 rad.

Gray scale Term describing the property of an image display in which intensity is recorded as variations in brightness.

Half-life Time in which half the atoms of a particular radioactive substance disintegrate. Time required for a 50% decrease in radioactivity.

Half-value layer (HVL) Thickness of absorber necessary to reduce an x-ray beam to half its original intensity.

Hard copy Permanent image on film or paper, as opposed to an image on a CRT, disk, or magnetic tape.

Health physics Science concerned with recognition, evaluation, and control of radiation hazards.

Hematopoietic syndrome (bone marrow syndrome) Form of acute radiation syndrome following whole-body exposure to doses ranging from approximately 1 to 10 Gy (100 to 1,000 rad) causing a reduction in circulating blood cells and a loss of the body's ability to clot blood and fight infection.

Hertz (Hz) Unit of frequency. Oscillations per second of a simple harmonic motion.

High-pass filter Convolution filter that suppresses the resolution of low-contrast tissue (liver) and enhances the resolution of high-contrast tissue (bone edges).

High-radiation area Area accessible to individuals in which radiation levels could exceed 100 mrem (1 mSv) in 1 hour.

Highly differentiated cells Mature or more specialized cells.

Homeostasis a. State of equilibrium among tissue and organs. b. Ability of the body to return to normal function despite infection and environmental changes.

Hormones Proteins manufactured by various endocrine glands and carried by the blood to regulate body functions such as growth and development.

Hydrocephaly Abnormal fluid in the brain.

Hydrogen peroxide (H_2O_2) Cellular poison that can result from the radiolysis of water.

Hydroperoxyl radical (HO_2) Substance toxic to the cell that can result from the radiolysis of water.

Hypoxia Lack of an adequate amount of oxygen.

Image intensifier Electronic vacuum tube that increases the brightness of a fluoroscopic image.

Image receptor Radiographic film or phosphorescent screen.

Impedance (See Acoustic impedance).

Incoherent scattering (See Compton scattering).

Indirect effect Molecular changes that result when a specific molecule such as DNA is acted on by free radicals previously produced by the interaction of radiation with water.

Inelastic scatter X-ray interaction with a loosely bound outer-shell electron resulting in a change in direction and a loss of energy.

Inertia Property of matter that resists its changing while in motion or at rest.

Infrared radiation Electromagnetic radiation just lower in energy than visible light with a wavelength in the range of 0.7 to 1,000 μm.

Inherent filtration Filtration of useful x-ray beam provided by the permanently installed components of an x-ray tube housing assembly and the glass window of an x-ray tube.

Ion Atom with too many or too few electrons, causing it to be chemically active or a free electron.

Ion pair Two oppositely charged particles.

Ionization Removal of an electron from an atom.

Ionization chamber Instrument that detects and measures radiation exposure by the electric current that flows when radiation ionizes gas in a chamber.

Ionize To remove an electron from an atom.

Ionizing radiation Radiation capable of ionization.

Ions Negatively and positively charged particles.

Insulator Material that inhibits the flow of electrons in a conductor or in heat transfer.

Interface Boundary between tissues having different ultrasonic properties.

Interference Phenomenon in which two or more waves of similar frequency add together or cancel each other according to their amplitude and phases.

Internal dose Portion of the dose equivalent received from radioactive material taken into the body.

International System of Units (SI) Standard system of units based on the meter, kilogram, and second adopted by all countries and used in all branches of science.

Interphase Period of cell growth that occurs between cell divisions.

Interphase death Death of a cell before the cell attempts division.

Inverse square law Law stating that the intensity of the radiation at a location is inversely proportional to the square of its distance from the source of radiation.

Irradiation Exposure to ionizing radiation.

Isobar Atoms having the same number of nucleons but different numbers of neutrons and protons.

Isomer Atoms having the same number of neutrons and protons but a different energy state of the nucleus.

Isotone Atoms having the same number of neutrons.

Isotope Atoms having the same number of protons.

Isotropic Equal intensity in all directions. Having the same properties in all directions.

Joule (J) Unit of energy. The work done when a force of 1 N acts on an object along a distance of 1 m.

Kerma (k) Energy absorbed per unit mass from the initial kinetic energy released in matter of all the electrons liberated by x or γ rays. Expressed in gray (Gy).1 Gy = 1 J/kg.

Kiloelectron volt (keV) The kinetic energy of an electron equivalent to 1,000 eV. 1 keV = 1,000 eV.

Kilogram (kg) 1,000 g.

Kilovolt (kV) Electric potential equal to 1,000 V.

Kinetic energy Energy of motion.

Laser Acronym for light amplification from stimulated emission of radiation.

Late effects Effects that appear months or years after exposure to ionizing radiation.

Latent period Period after the prodromal stage of the acute radiation syndrome during which there are no visible signs or symptoms of radiation exposure.

Lateral resolution Minimum separation of reflectors in a plane perpendicular to an ultrasound beam axis that can be distinguished.

Law of Bergonié and Tribondeau The radiosensitivity of cells is directly proportional to their reproductive activity and inversely proportional to their degree of differentiation.

LD$_{50/60}$ Dose of radiation expected to cause death within 60 days to 50% of those exposed.

Lead equivalent Thickness of radiation-absorbing material that produces an attenuation equivalent to that produced by a specified amount of lead.

Leakage radiation Secondary radiation emitted through x-ray tube housing. Does not include the useful beam.

Leukemia Neoplastic overproduction of white blood cells.

Leukemogenesis Origin or production of leukemia.

Leukocytes White blood cells.

Life-span shortening Shortening of life as a result of premature aging and disease.

Linear energy transfer (LET) Measure of the ability of energy transfer to biological material. Expressed in keV/μm of soft tissue.

Lipids Water-insoluble organic macromolecules that store energy for the body and consist only of carbon, hydrogen, and oxygen.

Liquid coupling Technique using a liquid such as gel or water to couple an ultrasound transducer to a patient.

Longitudinal wave Simple harmonic wave motion where the motion in the medium is in the direction of the wave (e.g., diagnostic ultrasound).

Low-pass filter Mathematical filter that suppresses the resolution of high-frequency structures (bone edges) and enhances the resolution of low-frequency structures (liver or spleen).

Lymphocyte White blood cell that plays an active role in providing immunity for the body by producing antibodies. Lymphocytes are the most radiosensitive blood cells.

M mode (motion mode) Method of ultrasound image display in which tissue depth is displayed on one axis and time is displayed along the second axis. M mode is used frequently to display echocardiographic signals.

Macromolecule Large molecule built from smaller chemical structures.

Magnetic dipole Current flowing in an infinitesimally small loop.

Magnetic dipole moment Vector with a magnitude equal to the product of the current flowing in a loop and the area of the current loop.

Magnetic flux density Oscillating electric and magnetic fields. A vector field quantity that results in a force acting on a moving charge. Also termed **magnetic field intensity**.

Magnetic permeability Property of a material causing it to attract the imaginary lines of the magnetic field.

Magnetic susceptibility Ease with which a substance can be magnetized.

Magnetization Relative magnetic flux density in a material compared with that in a vacuum.

Manifest illness Stage of the acute radiation syndrome during which signs and symptoms are apparent.

Manmade radiation X-rays and artificially produced radionuclides for nuclear medicine.

mAs (See Milliampere seconds).

Mass Quantity of matter (measured in kg).

Mass number (A) The number of nucleons (neutrons and protons) in the nucleus of an atom.

Matrix Rows and columns of pixels displayed on a digital image.

Matter Anything that occupies space and has form or shape.

Mean energy Average energy of an x-ray beam.

Mean marrow dose (MMD) Dose of radiation averaged over the entire active bone marrow.

Mega- Prefix that multiplies a basic unit by 1,000,000 or 10^6.

Megahertz One million cycles per second. 10^6 Hz.

Meiosis Process of germ cell division that reduces the chromosomes in each daughter cell to half the number of chromosomes in the parent cell.

Metaphase Phase of cell division during which the chromosomes are visible.

Micro- Prefix that divides a basic unit into 1 million parts or 10^{-6}.

Milli- Prefix that divides a basic unit by 1,000 or 10^{-3}.

Milliampere (mA) Measure of x-ray tube current.

Milliampere seconds (mAs) Product of exposure time and x-ray tube current. A measure of the total number of electrons.

Mitochondria Large bean-shaped structures containing highly organized enzymes in their inner membrane which function as "powerhouses" of the cell.

Mitosis Process of somatic cell division wherein a parent cell divides to form two daughter cells identical to the parent cell.

Mitotic delay Failure of a cell to start dividing on time.

Molecule Group of atoms of various elements held together by chemical forces. A molecule is the smallest unit of a compound that can exist by itself and retain all its chemical properties.

Monochromatic Having a single wavelength, as in the case of laser light.

Monoenergetic X or γ rays having a single energy.

Multiplanar reformation Use of the original transverse images to produce images in another body plane.

Mutations Changes in genes.

Myeloblasts White blood stem cells.

Nano- Prefix that divides a basic unit by 1 billion or 10^{-9}.

Natural background radiation (See Background radiation).

Near field Region of ultrasound beam lying between the transducer and the approximate focal depth.

Neutron Uncharged elementary particle, with a mass slightly greater than that of the proton, found in the nucleus of every atom heavier than hydrogen and in the nucleus of an atom.

Neutrophils Type of leukocyte that plays a role in fighting infection.

Newton Unit of force in the SI system. One newton corresponds to approximately 1/4 lb.

Noise a. Grainy or uneven appearance of an image caused by an insufficient number of primary x rays. b. Uniform signal produced by scattered x rays.

Nonoccupational exposure Radiation exposure received by members of the general public.

Nonstochastic effects Biological effects of ionizing radiation that demonstrate the existence of a threshold. The severity of the biological damage increases with increased dose. Also called **deterministic effects**.

Nonthermal effect Change in a medium or system that is not directly associated with heat when energy is absorbed.

NORM Naturally occurring radioactive material.

Nuclear fission (See Fission).

Nuclear force Powerful shortranged attractive force that holds nucleons together.

Nuclear fusion (See Fusion).

Nuclear reactor Mechanism for creating and continuing a controlled nuclear fission reaction for the production of energy and radionuclides.

Nuclear Regulatory Commission (NRC) (Formerly known as the Atomic Energy Commission [AEC].) Federal agency that enforces radiation protection standards.

Nucleic acids Large, complex macromolecules made up of nucleotides.

Nucleon Name for the two constituent particles of the atomic nucleus—neutrons and protons.

Nucleotides Units formed from a nitrogenous base (such as adenine, cytosine, deoxyribose guanine, or thymine), a five-carbon sugar molecule, and a phosphate molecule.

Nucleus a. Center of a living cell. A spherical mass of protoplasm containing the genetic material (DNA) which is stored in its molecular structure. b. Center of an atom containing neutrons and protons.

Nuclide General term referring to all known isotopes, both stable and unstable, of chemical elements.

Occupancy factor (T) Factor used to indicate the fraction of time that an area is likely to be occupied by a given individual.

Occupational dose Dose received by an individual in a restricted area or during the course of employment in which the individual's assigned duties involve exposure to radiation.

Occupational exposure Radiation exposure received by radiation workers.

Off-focus radiation X-rays emitted from parts of an anode other than the focal spot.

Oogonium Female germ cell.

Organic compounds All carbon biochemical compounds.

Organogenesis Period of gestation from the second to the eighth week after conception during which the nerve cells in the brain and spinal cord of the fetus develop and the fetus is most susceptible to radiationinduced congenital abnormalities.

Osteogenic sarcoma Bone cancer.

Osteoporosis Decalcification of bone.

Oxidation Combining of a substance with oxygen.

Pair production Interaction between an x ray of at least 1.02 MeV and the nucleus of an atom. The x ray disappears and two new particles, a negatron and a positron, are formed.

Partial volume effect Distortion of the signal intensity from a tissue because it extends partially into an adjacent slice thickness.

Particulate radiation As distinct from x and γ rays, examples are α particles, electrons, neutrons, and protons.

Penetrability Ability of x rays to penetrate tissue. Range in tissue. X-ray quality.

Personnel monitoring Determination of occupational radiation exposure by means of dosimetry.

Phantom Device that simulates some parameters of the human body for evaluating imager performance.

Photoelectric absorption Interaction between an x ray and an atom in which the x ray ceases to exist and an electron is ejected from its inner shell.

Photoelectron Electron ejected during the process of photoelectric absorption.

Photon Electromagnetic radiation that has neither mass nor electric charge but interacts with matter as though it is a particle. X rays and γ rays.

Pico- Prefix that divides a basic unit by 1 trillion or 10^{-12}.

Piezoelectric effect The property, exhibited by electrically asymmetric crystals, of generating electric potentials when mechanically stressed. Conversely, these crystals change size when electrically stressed.

Pixel Picture element of a digital image.

Platelets Circular or oval disks found in the blood that initiate blood clotting and prevent hemorrhage.

Pocket ionization chamber (pocket dosimeter) Personnel monitoring device.

Point mutations Genetic mutations in which the chromosome is not broken but the DNA within it is damaged by the breaking of a single chemical bond.

Polyenergetic Describes radiation such as x rays having many energies. Refers to a spectrum of energies.

Positive beam limitation (PBL) Feature of radiographic collimators that automatically adjusts the radiation field to the size of the image receptor.

Positron Unstable particle equal in mass, but opposite in charge, to the electron. A positive β particle.

Potential difference Difference in voltage between two points in a circuit.

Power Rate at which work is done. The rate of change in energy with time. Expressed in watts (W). 1 W = 1 J/s.

Primary beam (See Primary radiation).

Primary protective barrier Barrier in the line of travel of a primary x-ray beam.

Primary radiation X rays that emerge from an x-ray tube target

confined by collimation to the area of anatomical interest.

Prodrome First stage of the acute radiation syndrome which occurs within hours after radiation exposure.

Prophase Phase of cell division during which the nucleus and the chromosomes enlarge and the DNA begins to take structural form.

Protective apparel Items of clothing (i.e., aprons, gloves) that attenuate x rays to provide radiation protection.

Protective barrier Barrier of radiation-absorbing material used to reduce radiation exposure.

Protective housing Lead-lined metal container in which an x-ray tube is positioned.

Protein Amino acids that link together in various combinations and patterns.

Protocol Procedure to be used when performing a quality control measurement or related operation.

Proton Elementary particle with a positive electric charge equal to that of an electron and a mass approximately equal to that of a neutron. Located in the nucleus of an atom.

Protoplasm Building material of all living things.

Pulse average intensity (PA) Time average of ultrasound intensity over the pulse length.

Pulse length (PL) Time interval during which an ultrasound pulse is present. Also called **pulse duration**.

Pulse repetition frequency (PRF) Rate at which ultrasound pulses are produced. The inverse of the pulse repetition period, typically in the range 1.5 to 5 kHz. Also called **pulse repetition rate**.

Pulse repetition period (PRP) Time interval between the same point on an ultrasound waveform of two successive pulses.

Quality assurance All planned and systematic actions necessary to pro-

vide adequate confidence that a facility, system, or administrative component will perform safely and satisfactorily in service to a patient. Includes scheduling, preparation, and promptness in the examination or treatment and reporting the results, as well as quality control.

Quality control Included in quality assurance, comprises all actions necessary to control and verify the performance of equipment.

Quality factor (Q) (See Radiation weighting factor).

Quantum mottle Faint blotches on the radiographic image produced by fluctuation in the incident x-ray intensity. This effect is more noticeable when using very high rare-earth systems at high kVp.

Quantum theory Physics of electromagnetic radiation and of matter smaller than an atom.

Rad (radiation absorbed dose) Special unit for absorbed dose and air kerma. 1 rad = 100 erg/g = 0.01 Gy.

Radiation biology Branch of biology concerned with the effects of ionizing radiation on living systems.

Radioactive decay Naturally occurring process whereby an unstable atomic nucleus relieves its instability through the emission of one or more energetic particles.

Radiation detection instrument Device that detects and measures ionizing radiation.

Radiation hormesis Beneficial consequence of radiation for populations continuously exposed to low levels of radiation.

Radiation monitoring device Device worn by diagnostic radiology personnel to measure occupational exposure.

Radiation protection Techniques and tools employed by radiation workers to protect patients and personnel from exposure to ionizing radiation.

Radiation quality Relative penetrability of an x-ray beam determined by its average energy. Usually indicated by HVL or kVp.

Radiation quantity Intensity of radiation, usually measured in mR.

Radiation safety officer (RSO) Qualified individual designated by an institution to ensure that accepted guidelines for radiation protection are followed.

Radiation standards Recommendations, rules, and regulations regarding permissible concentrations, safe handling, techniques, transportation, industrial control, and control of radioactive material.

Radiation survey instruments Area monitoring devices that detect and/or measure radiation.

Radiation (thermal) Transfer of heat by emission of infrared electromagnetic radiation.

Radiation warning symbol Officially prescribed symbol (a magenta trefoil on a yellow background) that must be displayed where certain quantities of radioactive materials are present or where certain doses of radiation could be received.

Radiation weighting factor (W_R) Factor used for radiation protection purposes that accounts for differences in biological effectiveness between different radiations. Formerly called **quality factor**.

Radicals Groups of atoms that remain together during a chemical change, behaving almost like a single atom.

Radioactive Exhibiting radioactivity or pertaining to radioactivity.

Radioactive decay Decrease in amount of radioactivity with time as a result of spontaneous disintegration.

Radioactive half-life Time required for a radioisotope to decay to one-half its original activity.

Radioactivity Rate of decay or disintegration of radioactive material.

Expressed in curie (Ci) and becquerel (Bq). 1 Ci = 3.7×10^{10} Bq.

Radio frequency (RF) Electromagnetic radiation having frequencies from 0.3 kHz to 300 GHz.

Radiograph Image receptor, usually film, on which an image is created directly by an x-ray pattern and results in a permanent record.

Radiographer Individual who performs or personally supervises radiographic operations. A person qualified through formal education and certification to practice medical radiography.

Radiographic contrast Differences in optical density on a radiograph. Shades of gray.

Radiographic grid Device made of parallel radiopaque lead strips alternated with radiolucent strips of aluminum, plastic, or wood. It is placed between a patient and an image receptor to remove scattered x rays.

Radiographic intensifying screen Phosphor that increases the brightness of an x-ray image by converting it to a light image which then exposes the film.

Radioisotope Radioactive atoms having the same number of protons. They change into another atomic species by disintegration of the nucleus accompanied by the emission of ionizing radiation.

Radiological Society of North America (RSNA) Scientific society of radiologists and medical physicists.

Radiologist Qualified physician who specializes in medical imaging using x rays, ultrasound, and MRI.

Radiology Branch of medicine dealing with diagnostic and therapeutic applications of radiation in imaging or treatment.

Radiolucent Transparent to x rays.

Radiolysis of water Interaction of radiation with water.

Radionuclide Any nucleus that emits radiation.

Radionuclide (See Radioisotope).

Radiosensitivity Relative susceptibility of cells, tissues, and organs to the harmful action of ionizing radiation.

Radon Colorless, odorless, naturally occurring radioactive gas (^{222}Ra) which decays via α emission with a half-life of 3.8 days.

Random errors Errors that vary in a nonreproducible way around the mean.

Rayleigh scattering (See Classical scattering).

Real time Display for which the image is continuously renewed, often to view anatomical motion, fluoroscopy, and ultrasound.

Recessive mutation Genetic mutation that will probably not be expressed for a number of generations because both parents must possess the same mutation.

Reconstruction Creating an image from data.

Reflected wave Produced when an ultrasound beam in tissue is redirected by a discontinuity or an interface with a different tissue.

Reflection Reversal of the direction of an ultrasound beam when it encounters an extended interface with another tissue of different acoustic impedance.

Refraction a. Change in direction as an obliquely incident ultrasound beam travels from a tissue of one acoustic impedance to another tissue of differing acoustic impedance. b. Change in direction of visible light when traveling from one medium to another as seen at the air-water interface of a straw in a glass.

Region of interest (ROI) Area of anatomy on a reconstructed digital image as defined by the operator using a cursor.

Relative biological effectiveness (RBE) Relative ability of radiations with various LET values to produce a particular biological reaction.

Relative risk Refers to assumption that exposure to radiation will end in a steady percentage increase in cancers over the normal risk of malignancy occurring in people of all ages.

Relaxation a. Processes by which ultrasound energy is absorbed in a medium. b. Loss of tissue magnetization and return to equilibrium during MRI.

Relaxation time Time required for longitudinal or transverse tissue magnetization to return to equilibrium. Expressed in milliseconds (ms).

Rem (radiation equivalent man) Special unit for dose equivalent and effective dose. Replaced by the sievert (Sv) in the SI system. 1 rem = 0.01 Sv.

Remnant radiation All x rays that pass through a patient and interact with the image receptor.

Reproducibility (See Exposure reproducibility).

Reproductive cells Male and female germ cells.

Reproductive death Loss of the ability of a cell to reproduce, resulting from exposure to a moderate dose of ionizing radiation (100 to 1,000 rad).

Resolution Measure of the ability of a system to image two closely spaced structures.

Reverberation Phenomenon of multiple ultrasound reflections at tissue boundaries. Echoes are misplaced on the image, thereby presenting false information.

Ribonucleic acid (RNA) Type of nucleic acid that carries genetic information from DNA in the cell nucleus to the ribosomes located in the cytoplasm.

Ribosomes Small, spherical cytoplasmic organelles that attach to the endoplasmic reticulum.

Roentgen (R) Unit of exposure to x and γ radiation. 1 R = 2.58 × 10^{-4} C/kg.

Safe industries Industries that have an associated annual fatality accident rate of 1 or less per 10,000 workers (i.e., an average annual risk of 10^{-4}).

Sagittal plane Any anterior-posterior plane parallel to the long axis of the body.

Scalar Quantity or measurement that has only magnitude, as opposed to vector.

Scan Movement of an ultrasound or x-ray (CT) beam to produce an image. Change in magnetic fields and RF to produce an image (MRI).

Scanner Device to produce an axial or transaxial sectional image. Preferred terminology is **imager**.

Scattered radiation X rays that change direction after an interaction with matter. Classical and Compton scattering.

Scattering a. Process that causes ultrasound incident on irregular tissue boundaries or inhomogeneties to be changed in direction, frequency, phase, or polarization. b. Change in x-ray direction due to coherent scattering and Compton effect resulting in beam attenuation.

Secondary protective barrier Barrier that affords protection from secondary radiation.

Secondary radiation Leakage and scatter reaction.

Sector scan System of ultrasound imaging in which an ultrasound beam is rotated through an angle, resulting in a pie-slice-shaped image.

Sensitivity Minimum signal that can be detected.

Shadow shield Shield of radiopaque material suspended from above a radiographic beam-defining system to cast a shadow in the primary beam over the patient.

Shallow-dose equivalent (H_s) Applies to the external exposure of the skin or an extremity.

Shielding Material or obstruction that absorbs ionizing radiation and thus protects personnel or the public.

Side lobe Diffractive characteristic of an ultrasound beam in which secondary, off-axis intensities occur in the near or far field. Side lobes tend to limit lateral resolution.

Sievert (Sv) Special name for the SI unit of dose equivalent and effective dose. 1 Sv = 1 J kg^{-1} =100 rem.

Signal Information content of variation in current or voltage in a receiver.

Signal-to-noise-ratio (SNR) Sensitivity of a detector in recognizing a signal in the presence of background noise.

Sinusoidal Simple harmonic motion. A sine wave.

Skin erythema dose (SED) Dose of radiation (usually about 200 rad or 2 Gy) that causes redness of skin.

Solenoid Helical (spiral) winding of current-carrying wire that produces a magnetic field along its axis.

Somatic cells All cells in the human body with the exception of the germ cells.

Somatic effects Effects of radiation limited to an exposed individual, such as cancer and leukemia. Distinguished from genetic effects, which may also affect subsequent unexposed generations.

Sonar Acronym for sound navigation ranging.

Sonography Any imaging method using sound and yielding a graphical representation of tissue. This is a more inclusive term than ultrasonography.

Source-to-image-receptor distance (SID) Distance from a source (x-ray focal spot) to an image receptor (usually film or screen).

Source-to-skin distance (SSD) Distance between an x-ray tube target and the skin of a patient.

Spatial average intensity (SA) Intensity averaged over ultrasound beam cross-sectional area. Generally, this parameter is used when specifying the intensity for continuous-wave (CW) ultrasound.

Spatial average–temporal average intensity (SATA) Temporal average ultrasound intensity averaged over the beam cross-sectional area.

Spatial frequency Method of expressing size. A measure of the changes in tissue attenuation characteristics. Abrupt changes in tissue (e.g., at the bone-lung interface) have high spatial frequency, and gradual changes (e.g., at the liver-spleen interface) have low spatial frequency. Expressed in line pairs per millimeter (1 p/mm).

Spatial peak-pulse average intensity (SPPA) Value of ultrasound pulse average intensity at the point in a beam where pulse average intensity is a maximum.

Spatial peak-temporal average intensity (SPTA) Value of temporal average ultrasound intensity at the point in a beam where temporal average intensity is a maximum.

Spatial peak-temporal peak intensity (SPTP) Value of temporal peak ultrasound intensity at the point in a beam where temporal peak intensity is a maximum.

Spatial resolution Ability to image anatomical structures or small objects of high contrast.

Specific absorption rate (SAR) RF energy absorbed by tissue. An expression of dose of RF in MRI. Expressed in W/kg.

Spectrum Graphic representation of the range over which a quantity extends.

Speed of sound Product of the frequency (f) and the wavelength (λ) in tissue. Expressed in m/s. $V = f\lambda$.

Spermatogonium Male germ cell.

Spontaneous mutations Mutations in genes that occur at random and without a known cause. A natural phenomenon.

Standard Material or substance whose properties are believed to be known with sufficient accuracy to permit its use in evaluating the same properties of other materials.

Stem cells Immature or precursor cells.

Stochastic effects Probability or frequency of the biological response to radiation as a function of radiation dose. Disease incidence increases proportionately with dose, and there is no dose threshold.

Survey meter Portable device used for detecting radioactive contamination or measuring radiation exposure.

Systematic errors Errors that are reproducible and tend to bias a result in one direction.

Target a. Region of an x-ray tube anode struck by electrons emitted by the filament. b. The molecule-DNA-that is most sensitive to radiation.

Target molecule Molecule (DNA) that is few in number yet essential for cell survival and is particularly sensitive to the effects of ionizing radiation.

Target theory Theory that a cell will die if inactivation of the target molecule occurs as a result of radiation exposure.

Technique factors kVp and mAs as selected for a given radiographic examination.

Teletherapy Radiation oncology in which the source of radiation is at a distance from the body, as opposed to brachytherapy. Usually employs ^{60}Co.

Temporal average intensity (TA) The time average of ultrasound intensity at a point in tissue.

Temporal peak intensity Peak value of ultrasound intensity at the point in a tissue being considered.

Tenth-value layer (TVL) Thickness of absorber necessary to reduce an x-ray beam to one-tenth its original intensity. 1 TVL = 3.3 HVL.

Terrestrial radiation Portion of natural background radiation emitted by naturally occurring radioactive materials in the earth.

Tesla (T) SI unit of magnetic field intensity. An older unit is the gauss (G). 1 T = 10,000 G.

Test object a. Passive device that provides echoes and permits evaluation of one or more parameters of an ultrasound system but does not necessarily duplicate the acoustical properties of the human body. b. Passive device of geometric shapes designed to evaluate performance of x-ray and magnetic resonance imagers. (See Phantom).

Thermal energy Energy of molecular motion-heat, infrared radiation.

Thermal neutron Nominally classified as a neutron whose kinetic energy is approximately less than or equal to 1 eV.

Thermoluminescent dosimeter (TLD) Personnel monitoring device that most often contains a crystalline form (chips or powder) of lithium fluoride as its sensing material.

Thompson scattering (See Classical scattering).

Threshold dose Dose at which a response to an increasing x-ray intensity first occurs. Threshold dose may also be defined as a dose below which a person has a negligible chance of sustaining a specific biological response.

Thrombocytes (See Platelets).

Thymus gland Organ of the lymphatic system located in the mediastinal cavity anterior to and above the heart.

Thyroid gland Gland located in the neck just below the larynx.

Tissue weighting factor (W_T) Proportion of the risk of stochastic effects resulting from irradiation of the whole body when only an organ or tissue is irradiated.

Tomogram X-ray image of a coronal, sagittal, transverse, or oblique section through the body.

Total filtration Inherent filtration plus added filtration.

Tungsten Metal with a high melting point and high atomic number. Z = 74.

Transceiver a. Transducer used for both transmission and reception of ultrasound. b. Head or body coil when used to both transmit RF and receive a MRI signal.

Transducer Device capable of converting energy from one form to another. Specifically in ultrasound, the device used to convert electric energy to mechanical energy and visa versa.

Transition zone Portion of an ultrasound beam having no distinct boundaries between the near field and the far field.

Tritium Radioactive isotope of hydrogen (one proton and two neutrons). ^{3}H.

Ultrasound Acoustic radiation at frequencies above the range of human hearing, approximately 20 kHz.

Ultraviolet Electromagnetic radiation of a wavelength between that of the shortest visible violet and low-energy x rays.

Uncertainty Range of values within which the true value is estimated to lie.

Uncontrolled area Area in which members of the general public may be found.

Undifferentiated cells Immature or nonspecialized cells.

Unmodified scattering (See Classical scattering).

Use factor (*U*) Proportional amount of time during which an x-ray beam is energized or directed toward a particular barrier.

Useful beam (See Primary radiation).

Valence electrons Electrons in the outermost shell of an atom.

Variable aperture rectangular collimator Box-shaped device containing a radiographic beam-defining system. The device most often used to define the size and shape of a radiographic beam.

Vector Quantity or measurement that has magnitude and direction, as opposed to scalar.

Velocity of sound (See **Speed of sound**). The term velocity implies both direction and speed. The term speed of sound should be used where direction is of no concern.

Very high-radiation area Area accessible to individuals where radiation levels could result in their receiving an absorbed dose in excess of 500 rad (5 Gy) in 1 hour.

Visual acuity Ability to discriminate small image patterns.

Volt (V) SI unit of electric potential and potential difference.

Voltage Electric potential at a point or position relative to ground potential.

Waste, radioactive Gaseous, liquid, and solid materials from nuclear medicine procedures which are radioactive and for which there is no further use.

Wavelength Distance between similar points on a sine wave. Length of one cycle.

Weight Force on a mass caused by the acceleration of gravity. Properly expressed in newtons (N) but commonly expressed in pounds (lb).

Whole body For purposes of external exposure, head, trunk (including gonads), arms above the elbow, and legs above the knee.

Whole-body exposure Exposure in which the whole body rather than an isolated part is irradiated.

Window level Location on a digital image number scale where the levels of grays are assigned. Regulates the optical density of the displayed image.

Window width A specific number of gray levels or digital image numbers assigned to an image. Regulates the contrast of the displayed image.

Wipe sample Sample made by wiping a disk of filter paper over a surface for the purpose of detecting removable radioactive contamination. Also known as a smear sample.

Work Product of the force on an object and the distance over which the force acts. Expressed in joules (J). $W = Fd$.

Workload (W) Product of the maximum milliamperage (mA) and the number of x-ray examinations performed per week. Expressed in mA min/wk.

X-ray high-voltage generator Device that transforms electric energy from the potential supplied by an x-ray control to the x-ray tube operating potential.

X-ray imager X-ray system designed for radiography, tomography, or fluoroscopy.

X rays Penetrating ionizing electromagnetic radiation having a wavelength much shorter than that of visible light.

Yttrium Rare-earth phosphor used in rare-earth intensifying screens.

Appendix B

Appropriate Textbooks

Bushberg JT, Seibert JA, Leidholdt EMJr, Boone JM: The Essential Physics of Medical Imaging. Williams & Wilkins, Baltimore, 1994.

Bushong SC: Radiologic Science for Technologists—Physics, Biology and Protection, 6th ed. Mosby–Year Book, St. Louis, 1997.

Carlton RR, Adler AM: Principles of Radiographic Imaging—An Art and a Science. Delmar Publishers, Albany, NY, 1992.

Committee on the Biological Effects of Ionizing Radiations, Board on Radiation Effects Research, Commission on Life Sciences and National Research Council. Health Effects of Exposure to Low Levels of Ionizing Radiation—BEIR V. National Academy of Sciences, Washington, DC, 1990.

Dowd SB: Practical Radiation Protection and Applied Radiobiology: WB Saunders, Philadelphia, 1994.

Gurley LT, Callaway WJ: Introduction to Radiologic Technology, 3rd ed. Mosby–Year Book, St. Louis, 1992.

Hall EJ: Radiobiology for the Radiologist, 4th ed. JB Lippincott, Philadelphia, 1994.

Hendee WR, Ritenour ER: Medical Imaging Physics, 3rd ed. Mosby–Year Book, St. Louis, 1992.

Huda W, Slone RM: Review of Radiologic Physics. Williams & Wilkins, Baltimore, 1995.

Rosenbusch G, Oudkerk M, Ammann E: Radiology in Medical Diagnostics—Evolution of X-ray Applications 1895–1995, Blackwell Science, London, 1995.

Seeram E: Radiation Protection. Lippincott-Raven, Philadelphia, 1997.

Shleien B: The Health Physics and Radiological Health Handbook, rev. ed. Scinta, Silver Spring, MO, 1992.

Sprawls P Jr.: Physical Principles of Medical Imaging. Aspen Publishers, Gaithersburg, MD, 1993.

Thompson MA, Hattaway MP, Hall JD, Dowd SB: Principles of Imaging Science and Protection. WB Saunders, Philadelphia, 1994.

Statkiewicz MA, Ritenour ER: Radiation Protection for Student Radiographers. Multi-Media Publishing, Denver, CO, 1983.

Statkiewicz MA, Visconti PJ, Ritenour ER: Radiation Protection in Medical Radiography, 2nd ed. Mosby–Year Book, St. Louis, 1993.

Wagner LK, Archer BR: Minimizing Risks from Fluoroscopic X-rays—Bioeffects, Instrumentation and Examination. Partners in Radiation Management, Houston, TX, 1996.

Wagner LK, Lester RG, Saldana LR: Exposure of the Pregnant Patient to Diagnostic Radiations—A Guide to Medical Management, 2nd ed. Medical Physics Publishing, Madison, WI, 1997.

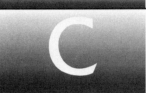

Answers

CHAPTER 1
1. b
2. d
3. d
4. a
5. b
6. b
7. a
8. d
9. b
10. d
11. b
12. a
13. b
14. c
15. d
16. d
17. c
18. d
19. d
20. c
21. a
22. b
23. b
24. d
25. a
26. a
27. c
28. c
29. b
30. c
31. c
32. a
33. c
34. d
35. d
36. b
37. c
38. b
39. a
40. d
41. a
42. d
43. a

CHAPTER 2
1. b
2. a
3. c
4. b
5. b
6. b
7. d
8. d
9. d
10. c
11. d
12. a
13. a
14. c
15. c
16. a
17. c
18. d
19. c
20. a
21. c
22. a
23. a
24. a
25. a
26. c
27. c
28. d
29. c
30. c

CHAPTER 3
1. c
2. c
3. a
4. d
5. a
6. a
7. a
8. d
9. b
10. d
11. a

12. b
13. b
14. b
15. a
16. a
17. d
18. b
19. c
20. b
21. b
22. c
23. a
24. c
25. c
26. a
27. d
28. c
29. c
30. c
31. d
32. d

CHAPTER 4
1. d
2. c
3. c
4. d
5. b
6. c
7. c
8. a
9. c
10. a
11. c
12. d
13. a
14. c
15. a
16. b

CHAPTER 5
1. a
2. a
3. c

4. d
5. d
6. b
7. c
8. c
9. d
10. b
11. c
12. c
13. d
14. d
15. d
16. a
17. a
18. a
19. a
20. d
21. d
22. c
23. b
24. b
25. b
26. a
27. c
28. b
29. d
30. a
31. c
32. a
33. b
34. b
35. c
36. c
37. c
38. d
39. a
40. a
41. d
42. c
43. b
44. c
45. c
46. b
47. b

48.	d	**CHAPTER 6**		56.	d	9.	c
49.	d	1.	a	57.	b	10.	c
50.	d	2.	b	58.	c	11.	c
51.	b	3.	d	59.	a	12.	c
52.	b	4.	b	60.	d	13.	d
53.	a	5.	b	61.	c	14.	b
54.	a	6.	b	62.	b	15.	b
55.	b	7.	d	63.	b	16.	a
56.	b	8.	a	64.	c	17.	a
57.	d	9.	b	65.	a	18.	d
58.	d	10.	c	66.	a	19.	a
59.	c	11.	b	67.	d	20.	a
60.	a	12.	c	68.	b	21.	a
61.	d	13.	a	69.	d	22.	b
62.	d	14.	c	70.	a	23.	a
63.	c	15.	c	71.	b	24.	d
64.	b	16.	d	72.	d	25.	d
65.	c	17.	b	73.	b	26.	c
66.	c	18.	a			27.	b
67.	b	19.	c	**CHAPTER 7**		28.	c
68.	b	20.	b	1.	b	29.	a
69.	c	21.	b	2.	b	30.	b
70.	d	22.	c	3.	d	31.	d
71.	b	23.	b	4.	a	32.	d
72.	d	24.	b	5.	d	33.	b
73.	b	25.	b	6.	c	34.	b
74.	d	26.	b	7.	c	35.	d
75.	a	27.	b	8.	d	36.	a
76.	b	28.	c	9.	d	37.	c
77.	b	29.	b	10.	d	38.	c
78.	b	30.	a	11.	b	39.	b
79.	d	31.	d	12.	b	40.	a
80.	d	32.	d	13.	c	41.	b
81.	c	33.	b	14.	a	42.	b
82.	b	34.	c	15.	b	43.	a
83.	b	35.	a	16.	a	44.	d
84.	b	36.	a	17.	c	45.	b
85.	d	37.	b	18.	d	46.	a
86.	c	38.	c	19.	d	47.	a
87.	a	39.	d	20.	c	48.	b
88.	c	40.	c	21.	d	49.	b
89.	b	41.	d	22.	a	50.	b
90.	b	42.	a	23.	c	51.	d
91.	b	43.	b	24.	d	52.	d
92.	a	44.	b	25.	c	53.	c
93.	b	45.	c	26.	c	54.	b
94.	b	46.	a			55.	b
95.	a	47.	a	**CHAPTER 8**		56.	b
96.	d	48.	c	1.	a	57.	b
97.	b	49.	d	2.	d	58.	c
98.	c	50.	d	3.	d	59.	a
99.	a	51.	a	4.	b	60.	a
100.	d	52.	c	5.	c	61.	b
101.	c	53.	a	6.	c	62.	a
102.	b	54.	b	7.	d	63.	a
103.	a	55.	b	8.	a	64.	b

65. d
66. d
67. d
68. d
69. d
70. d
71. d
72. d
73. c
74. d
75. d
76. c
77. c
78. a
79. a
80. d
81. c
82. b
83. d
84. d
85. b
86. c

CHAPTER 9 (Nuclear Medicine Imaging)

1. c
2. a
3. c
4. b
5. b
6. c
7. b
8. d
9. a

10. a
11. b
12. c
13. a
14. d
15. d
16. c
17. b
18. c
19. a
20. a
21. b
22. d
23. d
24. b
25. d
26. c
27. b
28. c
29. a
30. a

CHAPTER 9 (Diagnostic Ultrasound Imaging)

1. d
2. a
3. a
4. a
5. c
6. b
7. d
8. b
9. a
10. d

11. a
12. a
13. d
14. a
15. b
16. c
17. a
18. b
19. c
20. c
21. c
22. d
23. c
24. a
25. d
26. c
27. b
28. d

CHAPTER 9 (Magnetic Resonance Imaging)

1. c
2. b
3. d
4. c
5. c
6. b
7. a
8. d
9. a
10. d
11. a
12. b
13. a

14. b
15. c
16. d
17. b
18. d
19. d
20. c
21. d
22. d
23. d
24. d
25. a
26. b
27. b
28. a
29. d
30. c
31. c
32. a
33. b
34. a
35. b
36. d
37. d
38. b
39. c
40. d
41. d
42. c
43. d
44. b
45. b
46. b
47. b

Additional Resources

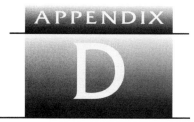

Access Publishing Company
1301 W Park Ave
Ocean, NJ 07712
Phone: 908-493-8811
Fax: 908-493-9713
Toll Free: 800-458-0990
E-mail: access@accesspub.com

American College of Radiology (ACR)
1891 Preston White Dr
Reston, VA 22091
Phone: 703-648-8956
Fax: 703-264-2443
Toll Free: 800-ACR-LINE

American Institute of Ultrasound in Medicine (AIUM)
14750 Sweitzer Ln, Suite 100
Laurel, MD 20707-5906
Phone: 301-498-4100
Fax: 301-498-4450
Toll Free: 800-638-5352
E-mail: membership@aium.org

American Registry of Diagnostic Medical Sonographers (ARDMS)
600 Jefferson Plaza, Suite 360
Rockville, MD 20852
Phone: 301-738-8401
Fax: 301-738-0312

American Registry of Radiologic Technologists (ARRT)
1255 Northland Dr
St. Paul, MN 55120-1155
Phone: 612-687-0048
Fax: 612-687-0449

American Roentgen Ray Society
1891 Preston White Dr
Reston, VA 22091
Phone: 703-648-8992
Fax: 703-264-8863
Toll Free: 800-438-2777
E-mail: ATTP:\\WWW.ARRS.ORG

American Society of Neuroradiology (ASNR)
2210 Midwest Rd, Suite 207
Oak Brook, IL 60521
Phone: 630-574-0220
Fax: 630-574-0061
E-mail: asnrsmit@interacess.com

Armed Forces Institute of Pathology (AFIP)
Dept of Radiology, Rm M121
Washington, DC 20306-6000
Phone: 202-782-2153
Fax: 202-782-0768

Churchill Livingstone
650 Avenue of the Americas
New York, NY 10011-2013
Phone: 212-206-5044
Fax: 212-727-7805
Toll Free: 800-451-6227

CRC Press, Inc
2000 Corporate Blvd NW
Boca Raton, FL 33431
Phone: 407-994-0555
Fax: 407-997-7249

Creative Educational Options, LLC
Thompson Nightingale International, Inc
553 Industrial Dr
2nd Floor, PO Box 537
Hartland, WI 53029-2342
Phone: 414-369-5838
Fax: 414-369-5842
E-mail: 7461.620@compuserve.com

Eastern Medical Publishers, Ltd
7455 New Ridge Rd, Suite Q
Hanover, MD 21076
Phone: 410-859-0400
Fax: 410-859-0480

Educational Reviews, Inc
6801 Cahaba Valley Rd
Birmingham, AL 35242
Phone: 205-991-5188
Fax: 205-995-1926
Toll Free: 800-633-4743

Educational Symposia, Inc
1527 Dale Mabry Hwy
Tampa, FL 33629-5808
Phone: 813-254-4608
Fax: 813-254-9773
Toll Free: 800-338-5901
E-mail: EDUSYMP@CYBERSPY.COM

Elsevier Science
655 Ave of the Americas
New York, NY 10010-5108
Phone: 212-989-5800
Fax: 212-633-3990

Harvard University Press
79 Garden St
Cambridge, MA 02138
Phone: 617-495-2650
Fax: 617-496-2550
Toll Free: 800-448-2242

Institute for Advanced Medical Education (formerly SONIX)
14 Elm Pl
Rye, NY 10580
Phone: 914-921-5700
Fax: 914-921-6048
E-mail: INFO@IAME.COM

International Commission on Radiation Units and
    Measurements, Inc
7910 Woodmont Ave, Suite 800
Bethesda, MD 20814-3095
Phone: 301-657-2652
Fax: 301-907-8767

International Society for Magnetic Resonance in Medicine
    (ISMRM)
2118 Milvia St, Suite 201
Berkeley, CA 94704
Phone: 510-841-1899
Fax: 510-841-2340
E-mail: INFO@ISMRM.ORG

John Wiley & Sons, Inc
605 3rd Ave
New York, NY 10158-0012
Phone: 212-850-6000
Fax: 212-850-6088
Toll Free: 800-225-5945
E-mail: HTTP://WWW.WILEY.COM

Lippincott-Raven Publishers
227 E Washington Square
Philadelphia, PA 19106-3780
Phone: 215-238-4200
Fax: 215-238-4227

Little, Brown and Co
34 Beacon St
Boston, MA 02108
Phone: 617-859-5543
Fax: 617-859-0629
Toll Free: 800-343-9204

The McGraw-Hill Companies, Inc
1221 Avenue of the Americas
New York, NY 10020
Phone: 614-755-4151
Fax: 212-512-2252
Toll Free: 800-262-4729

Medical Interactive
936 Dewing Ave, Suite D
Lafayette, CA 94549-4246
Phone: 510-283-7995
Fax: 510-284-1024

Medical Technology Management Institute (MTMI)
9722 W Watertown Plank Rd
PO Box 26337
Milwaukee, WI 53226-0337
Phone: 414-774-2233
Fax: 414-774-8498
Toll Free: 800-765-6864
E-mail: mtmi19@mail.idt.net

Mosby–Year Book, Inc
11830 Westline Industry Dr
St. Louis, MO 63146
Phone: 314-872-8370
Fax: 800-443-6106
Toll Free: 800-325-4177
E-mail: elva.walsh@mosby.com

MRI Education Foundation, Inc
2600 Euclid Ave
Cincinnati, OH 45219
Phone: 513-281-3400
Fax: 513-281-3420
Toll Free: 800-282-3404
E-mail: mri-efi@one.net

National Council on Radiation Protection and
    Measurements (NCRP)
7910 Woodmont Ave, Suite 800
Bethesda, MD 20814
Phone: 301-657-2652
Fax: 301-907-8768
Toll Free: 800-229-2652

Parthenon Publishing
1 Blue Hill Plaza
PO Box 1564
Pearl River, NY 10965
Phone: 914-735-9363
Fax: 914-735-1385
Toll Free: 800-735-4744

RSNA Membership Publications
2021 Spring Rd, Suite 600
Oakbrook, IL 60521
Phone: 630-571-2670
Fax: 630-571-7837
E-mail: http://www.rsna.org

Smart Charts
2047 University Blvd
Houston, TX 77030
Phone: 713-524-1509
Fax: 713-524-1509
E-mail: LHAYMAN@BCM.TMC.EDU

Society of Cardiovascular & Interventional Radiology
    Member Service
10201 Les Hwy, Suite 500
Fairfax, VA 22030
Phone: 703-691-1805
Fax: 703-691-1855
E-mail: INFO@SCVIR.ORG

Society of Diagnostic Medical Sonographers (SDMS)
12770 Coit Rd, Suite 508
Dallas, TX 75251
Phone: 214-239-7367
Fax: 214-239-7378
E-mail: sdms@sdms.org

Society of Nuclear Medicine
1850 Samuel Morse Dr
Reston, VA 22090-5316
Phone: 703-708-9000
Fax: 703-708-9015

Springer-Verlag
175 Fifth Ave
New York, NY 10010
Phone: 212-460-1500
Fax: 212-473-6272
E-mail: CUSTSERV@SPRINGER-NY.COM

WB Saunders Company
625 Walnut St, 300 East
Philadelphia, PA 19106
Phone: 215-238-7800
Fax: 215-238-8398
Toll Free: 800-523-4069

Williams & Wilkins
351 W Camden St
Baltimore, MD 21201-2436
Phone: 410-528-4000
Fax: 410-528-4305
Toll Free: 800-638-0672
E-mail: CUSTSERV@WWILKINS.COM
HTTP://WWW.WWILKINS.COM